# Feeding Your Baby
## Day by Day
✳ *From first tastes to family meals* ✳

## FIONA WILCOCK

LONDON  NEW YORK  MUNICH  MELBOURNE  DELHI

**Senior Editor** Claire Cross
**Designer** Harriet Yeomans
**Project Editor** Elizabeth Yeates
**US Editor** Christy Lusiak
**US Senior Editor** Shannon Beatty
**US Culinary Consultant** Kate Curnes-Ramos
**US Pediatric Consultant** Aviva Schein, MD
**Senior Pre-Production Producer** Andy Hilliard
**Senior Producer** Oliver Jeffreys
**Studio photography** Ian O'Leary
**Additional photography** Andy Crawford
**Managing Art Editor** Christine Keilty
**Publishing Manager** Anna Davidson
**Art Director** Jane Bull

DK INDIA
**Editor** K Nungshithoibi Singha
**Senior Editor** Charis Bhagianathan
**Senior Art Editor** Ivy Roy
**Art Editors** Zuarin Thoidingjam, Aparajita Barai
**Assistant Art Editor** Tanya Mehrotra
**DTP Designer** Sitish Gaur

First American edition, 2014
Published in the United States by
DK Publishing, 4th Floor, 345 Hudson Street,
New York, NY 10014

14 15 16 17 18   10 9 8 7 6 5 4 3 2 1
001 – 196666 – Feb/2014

Published in Great Britain by Dorling Kindersley Limited.

A catalog record for this book is available from the Library of Congress.

ISBN 978-1-4654-1595-0

DK books are available at special discounts when purchased in bulk
for sales promotions, premiums, fund-raising, or educational use. For
details, contact: DK Publishing Special Markets, 345 Hudson Street,
New York, New York 10014 or SpecialSales@dk.com.

Printed and bound in China by South China Printing Co. Ltd

Discover more at www.dk.com

# Contents

# Introduction

It's been nearly 20 years since my daughter was born, when the prevailing advice was to wait until four months to introduce any "solid" foods into a baby's diet, and then to opt for rice cereal. In the intervening years our understanding of both the science and psychology of feeding babies and children has improved, and the guidelines have changed alongside it.

However, in the work I do, and with the parents and babies I meet, I am still aware that whatever the guidelines are, this new stage in a baby's life can be a daunting time for parents, as they try to "get it right." Guidelines are, of course, written for populations, and each individual baby will have his or her own needs. In writing this book I have tried to unpack the science and psychology that are behind dietary recommendations by providing simple and practical advice and suggestions for parents. Where there are areas of debate I've included details so that you can make an informed decision about what you choose to do.

This book contains 200 fully tested recipes for the various stages and styles of weaning and these provide a progression of flavors and textures. So a parent starting with purées can try a host of delicious simple recipes from first tastes to more complex dishes, and a parent following a baby-led weaning approach will find plenty of nutritious suitable handleable foods for her baby. Whichever method you use, the aim is the same—to have your baby eating a wide range of nutritious foods and joining in with the family by the time her first birthday arrives.

I've devised menu plans from the first day of weaning right up to and beyond your baby's first birthday. These menu plans provide you with meals, ideas, and alternatives for each meal, making sure that each week your baby is exposed to new flavors and foods. They have been designed so that your baby has a great balance of different vegetables and fruits, learns to eat fish, poultry, and meat, enjoys dairy based meals and desserts, and tries different types of beans, grains, and potatoes. Foods that have been introduced in a simple form early on are repeated over the weeks, so that your baby has multiple exposures to nutritious foods, which evidence shows is a great way to engender good eating habits for life.

The menu plans have been devised to provide a wide range of nutrients to cover the needs of many babies. I don't claim that 100 per cent of the vitamin E your baby needs on any particular Tuesday will be supplied by that day's meals, as each recipe has not been individually analyzed for its nutritional content. However, I have used my experience as a nutritionist in feeding babies to put together the recipes and menu plans in a way which should provide great nutrition as well as enjoyable eating.

Of course, the menu plans don't need to be followed rigidly. They are there if you want clear guidance or may form the backbone of a weekly eating plan. However, you may prefer to use them for inspiration or ideas alone.

So I wish you fun as you start this exciting journey, introducing your child to the world of food, and hope that this book will help you on your way.

# *About* this book

**Feeding Your Baby Day by Day** starts with essential information on how to go about weaning your baby, then gives practical week-by-week meal planners followed by recipe sections organized by age and stage.

## Menu planners

There is a meal planner for each week of weaning in stages 1, 2, and 3. In the last section of the book, there is also a two-week sample planner full of ideas for family meals for the older ones. Every meal in the menu planners can be found in the recipe sections—cross references are given to help you to locate the recipes easily.

### Variations

In weaning stages 2 and 3, additional ideas for meals you could offer that week are suggested, to help you put together a week's menu that suits you and your baby.

*3¼in (8cm) diameter*

## Life-size bowls and spoons

Serving equipment is shown life-sized so you can see at a glance the approximate amount of food your baby should have per portion.

Stage 1

Stage 2

Stage 3

# Recipes

The recipe pages are ordered from light meals through to main meals and desserts, so it's easy to navigate your way around the recipes and reference this section independently of the menu planners if you wish.

There is no need to stop cooking recipes for younger babies once your baby has moved on to the next weaning stage. If your baby has some firm favourites, you can continue to cook these, simply adjusting the texture as necessary to suit your older baby.

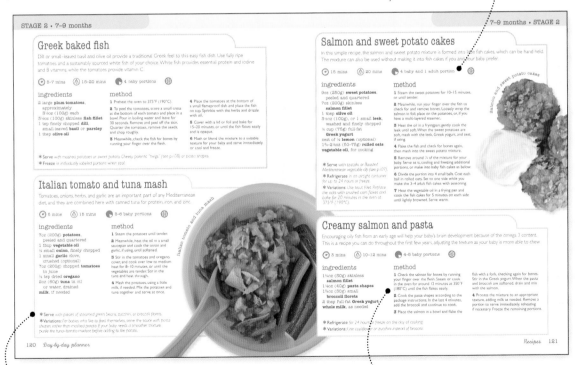

---- 5in (12cm) diameter ----

## Recipe Key

 Preparation time

 Cooking time

No cooking required

Number of portions

Suitable for freezing

## Portion sizes

For the more complex recipes, the number of both adult and baby portions is given, making it easier for you to share the meal with your baby.

*(recipe spread shown — page 120–121)*

STAGE 2 · 7–9 months

### Greek baked fish

Dill or small-leaved basil and olive oil provide a traditional Greek feel to this easy fish dish. Use fully ripe tomatoes and a sustainably sourced white fish of your choice. White fish provides essential protein and iodine and B vitamins, while the tomatoes provide vitamin C.

5–7 mins · 15–20 mins · 4 baby portions

**ingredients**
2 large **plum tomatoes**, approximately 3½oz (100g) each
3½oz (100g) skinless **fish fillet**
1 tsp finely chopped **dill**, small-leaved **basil** or **parsley**
1 tbsp **olive oil**

**method**
1 Preheat the oven to 375°F (190°C).
2 To peel the tomatoes, score a small cross at the bottom of each tomato and place in a bowl. Pour in boiling water and leave for 30 seconds. Remove and peel off the skin. Quarter the tomatoes, remove the seeds, and chop roughly.
3 Meanwhile, check the fish for bones by running your finger over the flesh.
4 Place the tomatoes at the bottom of a small flameproof dish and place the fish on top. Sprinkle with the herbs and drizzle with oil.
5 Cover with a lid or foil and bake for 15–20 minutes, or until the fish flakes easily and is opaque.
6 Mash or blend the mixture to a suitable texture for your baby and serve immediately or cool and freeze.

* Serve with mashed potatoes or sweet potato, Cheesy broccoli "twigs" (see p.138) or potato shapes.
* Freeze in individually labeled portions when cool.

### Italian tomato and tuna mash

Tomatoes, onions, herbs, and garlic are an important part of any Mediterranean diet, and they are combined here with canned tuna for protein, iron, and zinc.

5 mins · 15 mins · 6–8 baby portions

**ingredients**
7oz (200g) **potatoes**, peeled and quartered
1 tbsp **vegetable oil**
¼ small **onion**, finely chopped
1 small **garlic clove**, crushed (optional)
7oz (200g) chopped **tomatoes** in juice
¼ tsp dried **oregano**
2oz (60g) **tuna** in oil or water, drained
**milk**, if needed

**method**
1 Steam the potatoes until tender.
2 Meanwhile, heat the oil in a small saucepan and cook the onion and garlic, if using, until softened.
3 Stir in the tomatoes and oregano, cover, and cook over low to medium heat for 8–10 minutes, or until the vegetables are tender. Stir in the tuna and heat through.
4 Mash the potatoes, using a little milk, if needed. Mix the potatoes and tuna together and serve at once.

* Serve with pieces of steamed green beans, zucchini, or broccoli florets.
* Variations: For babies who like to feed themselves, serve the sauce with pasta shapes rather than mashed potato. If your baby needs a smoother texture, purée the tuna-tomato mixture before adding to the potato.

120 Day-by-day planner

---

7–9 months · STAGE 2

### Salmon and sweet potato cakes

In this simple recipe, the salmon and sweet potato mixture is formed into little fish cakes, which can be hand held. The mixture can also be used without making it into fish cakes if you and your baby prefer.

15 mins · 20 mins · 4 baby and 1 adult portion

**ingredients**
9oz (250g) **sweet potatoes**, peeled and quartered
7oz (200g) skinless **salmon fillet**
1 tbsp **olive oil**
3½oz (100g), or 1 small **leek**, washed and finely chopped
⅓ cup (75g) full-fat **Greek yogurt**
zest of ½ **lemon** (optional)
1¾–2¾oz (50–75g) **rolled oats**
**vegetable oil**, for cooking

**method**
1 Steam the sweet potatoes for 10–15 minutes, or until tender.
2 Meanwhile, run your finger over the fish to check for and remove bones. Loosely wrap the salmon in foil, place on the potatoes, or, if you have a multi-layered steamer.
3 Heat the oil in a frying pan, gently cook the leek until soft. When the sweet potatoes are soft, mash with the leek, Greek yogurt, and zest, if using.
4 Flake the fish and check for bones again, then mash into the sweet potato mixture.
5 Remove around ¼ of the mixture for your baby. Serve as is, cooling and freezing additional portions, or make into baby fish cakes as below.
6 Divide the portion into 4 small balls. Coat each ball in rolled oats. Set to one side while you make the 3–4 adult fish cakes with seasoning.
7 Heat the vegetable oil in a frying pan and cook the fish cakes for 5 minutes on each side until lightly browned. Serve warm.

* Serve with tzatziki or Roasted Mediterranean vegetable dip (see p.107).
* Refrigerate in an airtight container for up to 24 hours or freeze.
* Variations: Use trout fillet. Replace the oats with crushed corn flakes and bake for 20 minutes in the oven at 375°F (190°C).

### Creamy salmon and pasta

Encouraging oily fish from an early age will help your baby's brain development because of the omega 3 content. This is a recipe you can do throughout the first few years, adjusting the texture as your baby is more able to chew.

3 mins · 10–12 mins · 4–6 baby portions

**ingredients**
1½oz (80g) skinless **salmon fillet**
1½oz (40g) **pasta shapes**
1½oz (50g) small **broccoli florets**
2 tbsp full fat **Greek yogurt** or **whole milk**, as needed

**method**
1 Check the salmon for bones by running your finger over the flesh. Steam or cook in the oven for around 12 minutes at 350°F (180°C) until the fish flakes easily.
2 Cook the pasta shapes according to the package instructions. In the last 4 minutes, add the broccoli and continue to cook.
3 Place the salmon in a bowl and flake the fish with a fork, checking again for bones. Stir in the Greek yogurt. When the pasta and broccoli are softened, drain and mix with the salmon.
4 Process the mixture to an appropriate texture, adding milk as needed. Remove a portion to serve immediately, reheating if necessary. Freeze the remaining portions.

* Refrigerate for 24 hours or freeze on the day of cooking.
* Variations: Use cauliflower or zucchini instead of broccoli.

Recipes 121

## Serving, storage, and variations

Serving suggestions are provided at the end of recipes, as is guidance on cooling and how long food can be refrigerated or frozen. Recipe variations are also given sometimes, helping you to take account of seasonal availability and tastes.

## Oven temperatures

Temperatures are given in celsius, with fahrenheit conversions. If you have a convection oven, reduce the temperature by 50°F; for example, a recipe that requires an oven temperature of 375°F (190°C) would be 325°F (170°C) for a fan-assisted oven.

# Welcome to *weaning!*

Weaning your baby means starting to give her solid foods alongside her usual milk feeds. By the time your baby is a year old, she should be able to take part fully in your family meals. To find out everything you need to know, including when to start and what to do, read on.

# Is your baby *ready?*

**All babies grow and develop at different rates.** However, whether your baby was born early or late, struggled to establish breastfeeding, or sailed through the early weeks, there are some important developmental signs to look out for, usually present between four and six months, that indicate she is probably ready to start being weaned onto solid foods.

## Perfect timing

Working out the best time to wean your baby can make a difference to how smoothly the process goes. Most babies are weaned between four and six months; every baby is an individual and there is no one-size-fits-all rule as to when exactly to start your baby on solids. You do need to make sure your baby is showing the developmental signs shown opposite. Be guided by your baby and talk to your pediatrician if you're unsure whether she is ready, especially if she was premature (see pp34–35).

Never start weaning before four months of age. Before this age, your baby isn't able to process foods properly because her kidneys and digestive system are too immature. It's also inadvisable to leave it later than six months as by then your baby needs more nutrients than milk alone provides.

Continuing breastfeeding while weaning is thought to be beneficial, especially if you started weaning before six months. There is some evidence that babies who are breastfed alongside first solids (including allergenic foods such as wheat) before six months of age (but not before four months), are less likely to develop celiac disease, type 1 diabetes, or wheat allergy.

> *One of the main goals of the weaning process is to teach your baby to fit in with your healthy family meals.*

### What are the guidelines?

You may find yourself confused by contradictory official guidelines, as many governments advise exclusive breastfeeding for the first six months of life whenever possible. This advice stems from both the World Health Organization (WHO) and the American Academy of Pediatrics (AAP) due to the positive long-term effects of breast milk. The AAP recently recommended supplemental iron for exclusively breastfed babies (or babies who are mainly breastfed) over the age of 4 months if they are not taking any solids, because breast milk alone does not supply enough iron for babies this age. The recommended dose of iron is based on your baby's weight, so be sure to discuss with your pediatrician.

### A window of opportunity

When you decide to start weaning may be influenced by the so-called "window of opportunity." Child psychologists suggest that babies who are developmentally ready and start weaning between four and six months accept new tastes and textures more readily than those weaned later. This period, which extends to seven months, is seen as a chance to expand your baby's diet. If you wean at six months, you need to introduce new flavors more quickly, and move more rapidly on to lumps and finger foods.

**If your baby shows the following signs, she's probably ready for solids:**

### holds her head steady
Good head control is essential before your baby starts on solids; this muscular coordination also helps her swallow foods more easily.

### starting to chew
Your baby may start to make chewing motions, gnawing her fists and any other object that she picks up.

### shows an interest in food
She may be displaying a growing interest in what others are eating, and may even grab at the food on your plate.

### sits (maybe with support)
Your baby should be able to sit up before she starts weaning, although it's fine if she still needs some support.

### brings objects and food to her mouth
A willingness to explore everything with her mouth is one of the signs she's ready to wean; the first thing she may do with any new object is pop it in her mouth!

# Your baby's *changing* diet

**Milk dominates your baby's diet throughout the first year**, whether you are breast- or formula feeding, but by six months of age, her needs for growth and development are no longer met by milk alone.

Complementary, or weaning, foods are introduced to provide essential nutrients and different tastes and textures. Accepting new textures enhances your baby's learning of key skills such as chewing and speech development. As more foods are introduced and the quantity of these increases, some milk is naturally displaced, so what constitutes a balanced diet for your baby at 5 months will be different from her diet at 8 or 12 months, as solids become more

important. As your baby approaches one year, the amount of milk she drinks will have decreased from around 32oz (950ml) of formula or breastfeeding on demand, to 16–20oz (475–600ml) formula or two to three breastfeeds a day

Once your baby has gotten used to first tastes, she needs to eat foods from the same main food groups as you. However, the quantities and proportions are different to meet her high requirements for energy and nutrients.

## From milk to meals

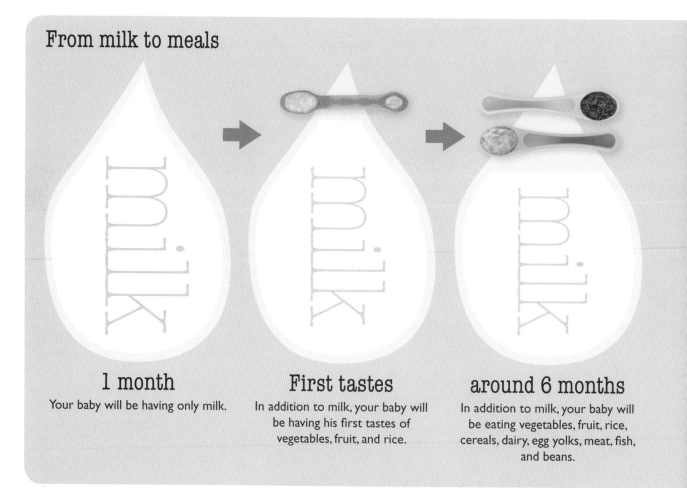

### 1 month
Your baby will be having only milk.

### First tastes
In addition to milk, your baby will be having his first tastes of vegetables, fruit, and rice.

### around 6 months
In addition to milk, your baby will be eating vegetables, fruit, rice, cereals, dairy, egg yolks, meat, fish, and beans.

## Milk and dairy foods

Full-fat milk, full-fat unsweetened yogurt and cottage cheese, and hard cheeses provide calories and protein as well as essential vitamins and minerals such as calcium, zinc, and magnesium.

## Bread, cereals, and potatoes

These starchy foods provide calories, B vitamins, and some iron. While whole-grain is good for adults, too much fiber can fill up your baby's tummy, not leaving enough space for other more nutritious foods. White bread, pasta, and rice are fine for babies; offer whole grains occasionally, gradually introducing more during the toddler and preschool years.

## Meat, poultry, fish, eggs, and beans

These foods provide protein, minerals, especially iron and zinc, fatty acids (from fish), and B vitamins.

## Vegetables and fruit

These provide vitamins, minerals, dietary fiber, and plant chemicals, sometimes called phytochemicals, such as antioxidants that protect the body from disease.

### 8 months
In addition to milk, your baby's diet includes all the food groups, provided in two to three meals each day.

### 10 months
The quantity of milk will be decreasing a little as your baby's diet includes more meals and larger portions of food.

### 12 months
Milk is still vital, but dairy foods play an important role, alongside iron-rich meat, fish, and poultry, cereals and potatoes, and vegetables and fruit.

# Food for *growing*

**Each food contains a mixture of different nutrients,** which have a range of functions to help your baby grow and develop. Some of the main nutrients that contribute to different areas of development are shown below. Some foods are especially good sources of particular nutrients, as shown on pages 16–17.

## For healthy growth:

**Protein** is the building block for every cell in your baby's body, and protein-rich foods are essential for her to grow and develop normally.

**Iron** forms part of the red blood cells that transport oxygen around the body. Too little iron causes anemia, which may cause delays in development and growth. By six months, your breast milk and the iron reserves your baby was born with no longer provide adequate iron, so providing iron-rich foods is important. In toddlers, anemia can be traced back to a poor weaning diet.

**Vitamin B2** helps keep skin healthy.

**Vitamin C** helps in the formation of blood vessels, muscles, cartilage, and bone.

**Vitamin E** is essential for the formation of red blood cells, muscles, and tissues, and helps keep skin healthy.

## For the eyes, brain, and nervous system:

**Omega 3 fatty acids** are essential polyunsaturated fatty acids for the development of your baby's brain, vision, and nervous system.

**Vitamin A** helps the healthy development of your baby's eyes.

**Vitamin B12** helps the development and working of your baby's nervous system.

**Folic acid** is essential for the nervous system and brain.

## For energy:

**Carbohydrates** Sugars and starch are carbohydrates that supply essential energy for your baby. Your baby doesn't need added sugars in her diet; sugars occur naturally in many foods including milk (breast milk is naturally sweet), fruits, and vegetables.

**Fats** are a concentrated source of energy (calories), which is perfect for your baby as she can eat only small amounts of food at a time. Around half of the calories in breast milk or formula come from fat, so it's important not to drop milk feeds when you start solids because your baby needs these for energy. As more foods are introduced, include small quantities of high-fat foods. Low- or reduced-fat foods aren't suitable for babies.

**B vitamins** help your baby release energy from carbohydrates and fats.

## For strong bones and teeth:

**Calcium** is essential for the healthy growth and development of your baby's bones and teeth. For the first few months, breast milk and formula supply this mineral, and although milk continues to be an important source, other calcium-rich foods need to be added to your baby's daily diet as you begin weaning, especially as the amount of milk gradually decreases.

**Vitamin D** has a wide range of protective roles and also works alongside calcium to help in the formation of your baby's teeth and bones. Babies who have inadequate vitamin D in the first year of life can develop the bone-softening disease rickets. As their bones aren't properly formed, this affects them when they start to stand or walk. Most vitamin D comes from the action of sunlight on the skin, and the body stores some for less sunny months. Rickets has started to recur in parts of the developed world as children spend less time outdoors exposed to sunshine. Very few foods contain much vitamin D, although some foods including infant breakfast cereals are now fortified with it.

**Vitamin A** helps strong growth in your baby's bones.

## For a healthy immune system and good healing:

**Zinc** is a mineral that helps promote growth, boosts the immune system, and helps wounds to heal, so including foods with zinc in your baby's diet in the first year is important. Most babies are not at risk of zinc deficiency, but if your baby was premature or is on a very restricted diet, talk to your pediatrician.

**Vitamin C** plays an important role in preventing infection as well as healing.

**Vitamin A** helps resist and fight infection. Some babies and toddlers don't have enough vitamin A, which makes them more prone to infections and other complications.

**Vitamin E** is an important, widely found vitamin that promotes healing.

# Know your *nutrients!*

**Each food your baby eats** is made up of various nutrients, including essential vitamins and minerals, so providing a range of healthy foods will help your baby flourish. The boxes below list the best sources of nutrients first. The meal planners in the book are designed to provide a healthy, balanced diet for your baby.

## Fats

| SOURCES | |
|---|---|
| | Oily fish, such as salmon, mackerel, and sardines |
| | Full-fat dairy: cheese, yogurt, and milk * |
| | Meat |
| | Oils, such as canola, olive, and vegetable |
| | Seeds and nuts (not whole) |

Fats are composed of a mixture of different types of fatty acids. Vegetable oils, seeds, and nuts contain more monounsaturated and polyunsaturated fatty acids, which are better for us than saturated fats, more commonly found in processed foods, dairy, and fatty meats. "Trans" fats, which are more likely to be found in lower quality processed food, are particularly unhealthy.

## Omega 3 fatty acids

| SOURCES | |
|---|---|
| | Oily fish, such as salmon, mackerel, and sardines |
| | Fish oil supplements [+] |
| | Nuts and seeds |
| | Vegetable oils |

The particularly good omega 3s are naturally present in fish oils. The other types of omega 3s from plant sources have to be converted in the body to the more useful type.

## Carbohydrates
### (includes starches and sugars)

| SOURCES | |
|---|---|
| | Bread |
| | Potatoes |
| | Rice and other grains |
| | Whole grains |
| | Fruits |
| | Vegetables |
| | Milk * |
| | Yogurt |

## Proteins

| SOURCES | |
|---|---|
| | Milk * |
| | Eggs |
| | Meat |
| | Poultry |
| | Fish |
| | Beans |
| | Tofu, quorn, or soy |
| | Nut and seed butters |

## Iron

| SOURCES | |
|---|---|
| | Canned sardines |
| | Liver ** |
| | Lean beef, lamb, and pork |
| | Dark cuts of chicken or turkey such as thigh |
| | Sausages |
| | Fish paste |
| | Fortified breakfast cereals |
| | Eggs |
| | Bread |
| | Beans, especially red kidney and navy |
| | Baked beans |
| | Tofu |
| | Dried fruit – prunes, figs, raisins, and golden raisins |
| | Cauliflower, broccoli, and spring greens |

There are two types of iron, one found in animal foods, the other in plant foods. Iron from animal sources is more easily absorbed. Vitamin C helps the absorption of iron from plant sources, so if your baby has little or no meat, try giving a cup of unsweetened fruit juice, diluted one part juice to 10 parts water at meal times.

## Calcium

SOURCES

- Hard cheeses, and soy "cheese"
- Canned fish (sardines or salmon)
- Tofu
- Milk *
- Yogurt
- White bread or products from white flour
- Dairy ice cream
- Beans, lentils, and chickpeas
- Squash and sweet potato
- Broccoli, spinach, and kale
- Peas
- Dates, golden raisins, and dried apricots

## Vitamin A

SOURCES

- Liver **
- Oily fish, such as salmon, mackerel, and sardines
- Fish oil supplements +
- Butter
- Egg yolk
- Carrots, sweet potatoes, mangoes
- Butternut squash, spinach, red pepper, andkale
- Cantaloupe melon
- Tomatoes, dried apricots, broccoli
- Pumpkin

## Vitamin C

SOURCES

- Red bell pepper, blackcurrants
- Strawberries
- Brussels sprouts, kiwi fruit
- Oranges, clementines, mangoes
- Nectarines, raspberries
- Grapefruit
- Papaya
- Cauliflower
- Rutabaga
- Cabbage
- New potatoes
- Pineapple, peas

## Vitamin B2

SOURCES

- Liver **
- Fortified breakfast cereals
- Cheese
- Almonds (ground)
- Milk *

## Vitamin D

SOURCES

- Oily fish, such as salmon, mackerel, and sardines
- Eggs
- Fortified breakfast cereals
- Butter and spreads

## Vitamin E

SOURCES

- Vegetable oils
- Nuts and seeds
- Avocado
- Eggs

## Vitamin B12

SOURCES

- Liver **
- Fish
- Meat
- Eggs

## Zinc

SOURCES

- Quorn
- Fish
- Meat
- Nut and seed butters
- Whole grains
- Eggs
- Milk *

## Folic acid

SOURCES

- Liver **
- Fortified breakfast cereals
- Broccoli
- Brussels sprouts and spinach
- Pinto and black eyed peas
- Beets, oranges

---

*   Don't use cow's milk as a drink before 12 months.
** Liver is so high in vitamin A, it is normally not recommended under one year. If given, this should be occasionally only.
+   Only use fish oil supplements that are suitable for babies and children, and not if you are using formula. Seek advice from your doctor.

# *Best* for baby

**Encouraging your baby to eat well from an early age helps her to grow** and develop into a healthy toddler and child, and has a positive long-term impact on her health and well-being. As well as making sure that your baby's diet includes different food groups that contain essential vitamins and minerals, getting her diet right is also about being aware of some other, often very particular, dietary requirements that apply to young babies.

## Avoid adding sugar unnecessarily

### Why?

Excess sugar in the diet can lead to tooth decay, and encourage your baby to develop a liking for sweet food over savory early on, which long-term could lead to obesity and nutrient deficiencies.

**What to watch out for:** If you breastfeed, up until weaning, your baby has been used to the sweet taste of your milk. As you start to introduce solids, it's important that she learns to accept savory tastes, so foods shouldn't be sweetened with sugar. Research also suggests that it's best if you don't mix sweet and savory foods either, so your baby learns to enjoy individual flavors.

Make sure that foods you buy don't contain added sugar. This can come in various guises including honey (which should be avoided before 12 months); sucrose, glucose, or fructose syrups; corn syrup; brown, cane, or beet sugar; and fruit juice concentrates, to name a few.

## White bread, pasta, and rice are fine for babies

Use whole-grain foods occasionally, and gradually introduce more during the toddler and preschool years.

### Why?

Foods that are full of fiber (which helps digestion and promotes good health), such as vegetables, fruits, and whole grains, tend to be quite bulky and don't provide much energy for your baby. This is great if you are a mom watching her weight, but bad news for a baby because her little tummy becomes full of low-calorie fiber, which doesn't provide enough energy or other nutrients for her to grow, and leaves less room for other more nutritious foods.

**What to watch out for:** Fruits and vegetables provide many essential nutrients, so it's a question of getting the balance right. Too many high-fiber foods can displace other nutritious foods such as dairy foods, meat, fish, eggs, and healthy oils. If as a family you eat only whole wheat bread, this is okay for your baby as long as she isn't having a lot of other fiber-rich foods such as lentils and beans.

> ## Never add salt to your baby's food
>
> Be aware, too, of hidden salts in other ingredients such as cured meats, smoked fish, brine-preserved ingredients, and high-salt cheeses.

## Why?

Too much salt at this age could also encourage a taste for salty foods, which could have negative effects later in life. Salt can overload your baby's developing kidneys, so it's important not to add any to her food. Salt is naturally present in many foods and your baby's requirements are more than met by these. Although her food may not taste as you would like it, it is perfect for her needs.

**What to watch out for:** Be cautious about using ingredients that are high in salt for family meals you are intending your older baby to share. If necessary, add ingredients such as bacon and cured meats, smoked fish, or olives and other brine-preserved foods to the main dish after her portion has been served and is cooling.

Look at ingredients on food labels and choose those lowest in salt. Use fish or vegetables canned in water or oil, not brine; avoid high-salt cheeses such as Parmesan; and buy salt-free tomato purées and pastes.

Savory snacks, such as pretzels and potato or corn chips are very salty and are unsuitable for babies.

## Not for babies

There are a few other foods that should be avoided in your baby's first year:

- Honey, due to the small risk of a food poisoning bacterium that can cause infant botulism
- Whole nuts because of the risk of choking
- Shellfish, due to the risk of food poisoning
- Shark, marlin, and swordfish, which may contain mercury or other potential toxins
- Liver, due to its very high vitamin A content
- Unpasteurized cheeses or dairy products
- Diet, or reduced fat or sugar, foods, or drink.

## Organic or non-organic?

Organic farms use fewer chemicals, but is organic food nutritionally better? Evidence is varied and depends on the type of food, the season, even how long a farm has been organic, but it's thought that mostly it doesn't provide more nutrients.

If you buy fresh organic food, bear in mind the shelf life is shorter and wash it carefully before use.

Products grown for commercial baby food are stringently regulated, and therefore there's little, if any, difference between organic and non-organic products.

## Do babies need vitamin supplements?

Supplements of vitamins A, D, and C are important for babies with a limited diet, fussy eaters, and for those who don't drink 16oz (475ml) of formula milk a day. The AAP recommends that exclusively breastfed babies or babies that take less than 16oz (475ml) of formula day get a Vitamin D supplement (400IU/day). Breastfeeding moms are advised to take a vitamin D supplement too.

# What's your *style?*

**The most usual method of weaning is to start with puréed foods,** gradually adapting textures and adding tastes. Another approach, known as baby-led weaning, concentrates on babies feeding themselves whole foods from the outset, starting at six months. Whichever method you follow, the aim is the same: for your baby to be eating healthy, balanced meals with the rest of the family by 12 months of age.

## Weaning with purées

For many cultures, weaning starts with giving a baby puréed food from a spoon. The texture of the food varies, starting with runny purées, progressing through to mashed food, food with soft lumps, soft finger foods, and then ground and chopped foods with harder finger foods. At each stage, your baby learns something new and develops new skills. The aim is that by one year she will be able to eat chopped versions of suitable family meals, have started to self-feed using a spoon and/or fingers, and be drinking from a cup (with or without a spout). She will have had the opportunity to try repeatedly a wide range of different foods from all the main food groups, and been part of family meals and social eating occasions.

> *During weaning, you introduce your baby gradually to the foods she will eat throughout her life.*

## Baby-led weaning (BLW)

This method promotes offering whole cooked foods or soft raw foods rather than puréed foods to your baby, and allows her to feed herself from the outset rather than being spoon-fed by you. BLW allows your baby to take the lead in deciding which foods to try when. It is often said to be a more relaxed, if messy, approach to weaning as babies can enjoy feeling, squishing, and playing with the food as well as eating it.

Advocates claim that it results in children being less fussy about food and better able to control their appetite, which may reduce their risk of becoming overweight, although this has yet to be confirmed by research.

## How do you choose?

There are pros and cons to both weaning methods. The more usual purée route is tried and tested, and research shows that it works nutritionally and developmentally. The danger is that babies may struggle moving from purées to lumps if kept on runny purées for too long.

Babies following the BLW route need sufficient hand–eye coordination to pick up food, which ties in with current recommendations to delay weaning to six months. However, there is less research on BLW, and claims that this approach reduces fussy eating later on are yet to be established. It is also not known if babies get adequate nutrition at first, especially of iron, so if you adopt this approach, you still need to ensure that your baby's diet is nutritious and balanced, rather than simply giving foods you happen to be eating.

Your decision may be influenced by your personalities and your baby's abilities. You and your baby may be temperamentally more suited to controlled purée feeding: she may prefer to be spoon fed until she gains more confidence, and you may appreciate the structure. Alternatively, if your baby has good hand–eye coordination and is independent, she may want to hold a spoon or a piece of food, so if you're happy with the extra mess of BLW, this may work well. There is no reason why you can't combine weaning approaches, or you may wish to try one or the other method first, then work out what suits you both best.

# As *easy as* 1, 2, 3...

**Weaning is usually described in three stages.** During each stage, as well as trying out new foods and textures, your baby develops new skills that help her to eat solids. She learns how to use her tongue, to swallow different textured purées, to chew up and down then in a rotary fashion, and to pick up food and move it to her mouth. She also learns to use her lips to move food from a spoon and to drink from a cup.

## Stage 1 — up to 7 months

In the first stage, your baby learns:

- to take food from a spoon by closing her mouth around it
- to move food from the front to the back of her mouth to swallow
- that foods taste different
- to accept purées and then mashed foods, and she may try some first finger foods

Runny purée

Thicker purée

Mashed food

## Stage 2 — from 7 to 9 months

In this stage, your baby learns:

- to move lumps around in her mouth
- to become confident chewing soft lumps
- to use a pincer grip to self-feed soft or dissolving finger foods
- to drink from a sippy cup
- to accept a wider range of different foods
- to eat more than one meal a day

Mashed food

Mashed food with soft lumps

Soft or dissolving finger foods

## Stage 3 — from 9 to 12 months

In this stage, your baby learns to:

- master chewing ground and chopped foods
- eat a greater number of finger foods including those with harder textures
- use her lips to get food off a spoon and become more proficient at self-feeding with a spoon
- curl her lips around a sippy cup
- accept a wider range of suitable family foods
- eat three meals a day

Finely ground or chopped food

Ground or chopped food with larger pieces

Harder finger foods

## Baby-led weaning

from around 6 months

- If you follow baby-led weaning, starting around six months, your baby will sit with you at mealtimes (whenever possible), and be offered a selection of whole cooked foods or soft fruit, cut into easy-to-handle pieces. She may simply play with the food at first, perhaps suck it, then gradually will start to chew and swallow food.

- If you wish to combine BLW with purée-based weaning, offer soft finger foods alongside purées at around six months.

- You can be led by the planner to ensure your baby receives a balanced diet, cooking and offering the meals chopped rather than puréed or mashed.

## Family meals

from 12 months onward

By 12 months your baby will:

- be eating chopped up versions of family meals

- be eating together with the family whenever possible

- be drinking from a lidded cup or sippy cup

Chopped up family meals

# Time to *shop*

**Once your baby starts on solids,** you will want to be sure that your shopping cart contains pantry basics that are suitable for her to eat. Thankfully, many family ingredients are fine for your baby, with just a few that aren't suitable. Knowing which items are okay and which aren't will help you shop with confidence and make the best choices for your baby.

**Cheese:** full-fat hard cheese for cooking and full-fat cream cheese for spreads and dips.

**Spreads:** full-fat made from olive or sunflower oil.

**Oils:** monounsaturated vegetable oils such as canola or olive oil.

**Yogurts and cottage cheese:** natural, full-fat, unsweetened varieties. Sweeten them naturally with homemade purées or stewed fruits.

**Cereals:** low sugar and salt varieties; iron-fortified.

**Frozen vegetables:** frozen vegetables, such as chopped spinach, peas, and butternut squash sometimes have a higher nutritional value than fresh versions as they are frozen at their peak condition.

**Milk:** full- or low-fat cow's milk can be used for cooking after six months. It isn't suitable as a drink before one year as it doesn't provide sufficient iron.

**Canned chopped tomatoes or tomato sauce:** useful when making family meals to share with older babies. Choose varieties with no added sugar or salt.

**Spices, herbs, ginger, and garlic.**

**Commercial baby foods:** there is a good range of commercial baby foods, with many providing a wide variety of ingredients and nutrients.

**Canned foods:** opt for fruits preserved in their juices; vegetables and beans in water; tuna in water or oil. Cans are convenient and offer a variety of colors and flavors when fresh fruit or vegetables aren't in season.

**Bread, pasta, and rice:** white varieties; some whole-grain is okay.

**Fruits and vegetables:** seasonal, in a variety of colors.

## Leave it on the shelf!

The following items shouldn't be included in your baby's pantry or diet.

- **Fruit juices** provide vitamin C, but they're high in sugars, which can lead to tooth decay and a preference for sweet food. Strictly limit or avoid these, unless your baby is a vegetarian, in which case giving unsweetened fruit juice diluted one part to 10 with water at mealtimes helps iron absorption.

- **Soft drinks** also encourage a sweet tooth and can cause tooth decay. Fizzy drinks and artificially sweetened diet drinks intended for adults should definitely be avoided.

- **Drinks containing caffeine** aren't suitable for babies or small children. Tea and coffee are stimulants and contain tannins, which affect the absorption of iron.

- Avoid **salty foods and sauces** such as soy sauce; tomato ketchup; spicy curry sauces; sauces with added cheese, ham, or bacon; chutneys and pickles; cured meats (bacon, salami); chips or other savory snacks; olives preserved in brine; adult frozen entrées, and boullion cubes.

- **Chili** isn't suitable for babies.

- Your baby doesn't need **candy or sugar**, unless used to sweeten a sour fruit when cooking, so avoid sweet processed foods such as jams, some breakfast cereals, cakes, cookies, ice-creams, and popsicles. Pudding is okay occasionally, but check that the color comes only from betacarotene and, if using powdered pudding, make it with a minimum of sugar.

- **Goat or sheep milk** can be allergenic and these don't provide sufficient nutrients for your baby under one year.

- **Butter** is high in saturated fat so should be used only sparingly.

# Into the *kitchen*

**With the right equipment and preparation,** making homemade purées is simple. You need to be scrupulous about kitchen hygiene and store food correctly to ensure it stays as fresh as possible. Build in preparation time for chopping and slicing fresh produce and think about quantities too: cooking more than your baby needs for one meal means you can freeze purées and have pre-made meals on hand for busy days.

## Safety first

Young babies are more vulnerable to infections than adults so it's vital that you follow good hygiene practice while preparing your baby's food to minimize the risk of transferring germs and infections to your baby.

- Wash your hands with soap before handling food.

- Before and after preparing and cooking your baby's food, wipe surfaces thoroughly with a clean cloth soaked in hot, soapy water to eliminate germs and bacteria. Use disposable cloths or rotate clean cloths daily.

- If you have pets, don't allow them on work surfaces or near foods. Use separate utensils and bowls for pets.

- Wash fruit, vegetables, and potatoes before preparing.

- Cook eggs until solid and meat and poultry until there's no pink flesh and the juices run clear.

## Preparing food

Making healthy homemade food for your baby involves quite a bit of preparation time as you peel, chop, and slice fresh produce. You may already have everything you need to do this, but it's worth making sure your knives are sharpened and cutting boards aren't too worn. If you wish, you might want to invest in equipment such as a food processor to help speed up the process; there is a range of models available depending on your needs.

### A sharp knife
A properly sharpened knife is a basic essential for efficient home cooking.

### Cutting boards
Use separate cutting boards for preparing raw items such as meat and fish, and cooked items or fruit and vegetables to prevent cross contamination.

### Mini chopper
Mini food processors chop small amounts of food quickly. Look for one with more than one speed that enables you to control texture.

### Food processor
These can have a variety of functions, including chopping and puréeing, and the cost varies accordingly. If you enjoy cooking, you might want to invest in a more expensive model with discs for grating and slicing.

# Batch cooking and freezing

Your baby eats only small quantities of food at a time, so batch-cooking and freezing larger quantities avoids wastage and reduces the amount of time you spend in the kitchen. Vitamins are lost during preparation and storage, so chill and freeze foods quickly to minimize losses.

 **Freezing:** Pour hot purées straight into ice-cube trays or small containers, cover, let cool thoroughly (not in the fridge), then freeze immediately. On a hot day, you can place food in sealed containers and pop these into a bowl of cold water with ice cubes to speed up chilling. Label the container or tray with the content and date and freeze at 0°F/-18°C.

**Defrosting:** The safest way to defrost foods is overnight in the fridge. They can also be defrosted in a bowl in a microwave following microwave instructions. Don't leave foods to defrost at room temperature, particularly if they contain meat or fish.

**Reheating:** Defrosted food can be reheated in the microwave (or a pan) until it is piping hot, then removed and stirred well to get rid of "hot spots." Cool the food before serving to your baby, checking the temperature by testing a blob on the inside of your wrist: it should feel neither hot nor cold. Cool it for a few more minutes if it's still hot. Reheat defrosted foods once only.

# Useful storage items

**Lidded plastic containers and ice-cube trays**
Lidded plastic containers are handy for storing items in the fridge, keeping them separate from other foods. Individual ice-cube trays or lidded portion containers or ice-cube trays are ideal for freezing purées as you can defrost just the quantity of ice-cube portions required for one meal.

## ⚛ Storing foods

**For the fridge,** follow these guidelines to keep fresh, perishable produce at its best:

- Set your fridge at 39.2°F (4°C). Use a thermometer if you wish.
- Keep the most perishable foods such as meat, fish, and poultry in the coldest part of the fridge.
- Raw foods such as meat, fish, and poultry should be well wrapped, or put in an airtight container so they don't drip on other foods.
- Loosely wrap vegetables and fruits in plastic bags.
- Check "use by" dates on foods that may spoil quickly, such as dairy, fish, and meat; these are unsafe to eat after this date. If a label states an item can be eaten within three days of opening but this passes the use-by date, it isn't safe to eat.
- Don't keep food that your baby has half eaten.

**In the pantry,** for non-perishable foods:

- Ensure the cupboard is cool and dry.
- Rotate foods so the first in are eaten first, and follow the instructions for storage on the label.
- Check "best before" dates on foods such as pasta, cereals, and rice. These foods aren't unsafe to eat after this date, but the taste or quality may decline. The exception is eggs, which should be eaten within a couple of days after the "best before" date.

# How to make *baby purées*

**Cooking baby purées is quite straightforward,** and you will probably find that you derive a great deal of pleasure from cooking nutritious food for your baby. Being well organized, for example ensuring that food is ready before your baby becomes too hungry and upset, will make mealtimes more relaxed. Make sure your ingredients are in peak condition and cook foods thoroughly to avoid food poisoning.

## 1 Cook the ingredients until just tender

Apart from a few fruits that can be given to your baby raw, most first foods need to be cooked to reduce the risk of food poisoning. Cooking destroys around half of the vitamin C content of food and some B vitamins (more if the water they are cooked in is thrown away), so when possible use methods such as steaming, which preserves the most vitamins and minerals. Sometimes, though, the nutrient content of a food actually improves with cooking. For example, the naturally occurring chemical lycopene, found in tomatoes, which has specific health benefits, is released more readily with cooking. Cooking also makes dietary fiber more digestible.

### Steaming

This is a good way to cook vegetables and potatoes as it's quicker than boiling and the food doesn't come into contact with water so fewer vitamins and minerals are lost.

### Oven baking

Some fruits or vegetables can be softened by oven baking, which is an economical cooking method if the oven is already in use.

### Stewing

Fruits such as apples and pears need to be softened by stewing them gently in a little water. The cooking liquid can then be added to the fruit when puréeing.

### Boiling

Pasta, rice, and other grains need to be boiled in salt-free water, then drained before being mixed with other ingredients and served.

**Meat and poultry** need longer cooking times to become tender, so stewing with vegetables in water or with salt-free stock is the best cooking method.

# 2 Transfer cooked food to the equipment for puréeing

In the early weeks of weaning with purées, you need to make sure that your baby's food is the right consistency after cooking (see below) before serving it to your baby.

You can strain the cooked food through a mesh strainer using a fork, or you might want to invest in some additional kitchen equipment to achieve a good purée.

## Equipment

Some equipment combines several functions, while other items have just one or two uses. It's easy to be overwhelmed by the choice, so think about your requirements before purchasing. Do you want something that produces food with different textures? Will you use it once your baby has passed the weaning stage? Is the equipment easy to clean and dishwasher friendly, and how much space does it take up?

### A mouli (food grinder)

This utensil pushes food through a rotating grating disc to produce a fine consistency. These are popular for potatoes, which become sticky in a blender or processor, but less commonly used for other foods.

### A masher or ricer

A masher is good for making slightly lumpier textures, as is a ricer, which acts like a press that forces food through different sized discs. Ricers have limited use, but are perfect for potatoes and root vegetables.

### An electric hand blender

This makes great purées and can also be used to blend soups and get lumps out of sauces. Some come with attachments and other useful blades. Blenders with more than one speed can produce different textures.

### Food processors, mini choppers, and blenders

Food processors can chop, slice, and purée; more compact mini choppers are also available. Models with different speeds help you control the texture of purées. A blender has fewer functions, but also purées well.

# 3 Blend until it is smooth

The consistency of first purées should be almost runny, similar to a non-set yogurt. If a purée is too thick, you can adjust the texture by adding your baby's usual milk or cooled boiled water. If it's too thin, add more of the food or a spoonful of baby rice. Meat and poultry are usually introduced a bit later in the weaning process when your baby is starting to eat lumpier food, which is helpful as the fibers are more difficult to process finely.

# Time to *eat*

**You've cooked and cooled your baby's food**, and now you're ready to serve. There are a few items that are well worth buying or borrowing to help your baby's mealtimes go smoothly, allowing you and your baby to concentrate on the job at hand.

## Serving your baby's food

**A secure feeding or high chair**
A supportive high chair with straps ensures your baby is safely seated for feeding. When choosing one, think about your available space, whether the chair is easy to clean and portable (does it fold away when visiting friends or family?), and does it have a removable tray if you wish to draw your baby up to the table?

**Bibs**
These save on endless changes of outfit. Soft fabric bibs are comfy for younger babies, and all-in-one overall bibs are ideal for babies who are finger feeding. Pelican bibs have a collection tray at the bottom to catch dropped food.

**Spoons**
You need plenty of soft, long-handled, flexible plastic weaning spoons, which are more pleasant for your baby to put in her mouth than hard metal.

**A lidded cup**
This can be introduced from six months. Your baby can start to drink water or formula milk from a lidded cup, which helps with hand–eye coordination and learning to swallow.

## Washing, sterilizing, and cleaning

- For babies under six months old, sterilize baby feeding spoons and bottles.
- After six months of age, wash your baby's food bowl and utensils in the dishwasher or in hot water and dry them with a clean kitchen towel.
- Clean your baby's high chair thoroughly after each meal, wiping away lodged food.
- Wash your baby's hands before she eats.

## Make a mess!

As your baby grows, she will naturally start to explore food with her hands, which can be a messy business! It's tempting to mop her up as she goes along, but letting her interact with her food is an important part of learning. As she touches, squishes, and smears, she is finding out about texture, size, temperature, and shape. She is also developing her motor coordination as she finesses her grasp then attempts to transfer food from hand to mouth, exploration that will eventually lead to successful self-feeding with a spoon. Each new experience is exciting to your baby, and allowing her to explore food on her own terms means she is more likely to accept new foods and avoid being a fussy eater later on. Putting a splash mat or old newspapers under the high chair limits the chaos at ground level!

# Is it an *allergy?*

**Parents are often anxious about how and when to introduce foods** that carry a higher risk of allergy to their baby's diet, and anxiety is fueled by conflicting advice, with the latest research sometimes contradicting official guidelines. More children are developing adverse reactions to food, and if your child suffers a reaction, this is alarming. Reassuringly, though, only a tiny proportion have serious or life-threatening reactions, and many children grow out of the most common allergies, to milk and eggs, by the age of five.

## Allergy or intolerance?

Both of these mean that a food has caused an adverse reaction in the body, resulting in a "hypersensitivity" to the food. In an allergic reaction, the immune system reacts abnormally to a food, triggering the release of antibodies to the protein in the food, usually resulting in immediate symptoms. An intolerance doesn't involve the immune system and can be harder to spot as symptoms are slower to develop and can be linked to other childhood conditions.

### *Should my baby avoid gluten?*

Wheat, rye, and barley contain the protein gluten. Some people are genetically susceptible to gluten and cannot process it, which can result in celiac disease, whereby the immune system treats gluten as a potential threat and attacks it, causing the gut to become sore and inflamed.

In the US, studies are inconclusive or still ongoing about when to introduce gluten. Some research recommends avoiding giving gluten-containing foods before six months. However, other research suggests that introducing it before six months (but not before four months) alongside breastfeeding may reduce the risk of developing celiac disease, type 1 diabetes, and wheat allergy. The best advice may be to continue breastfeeding while you introduce wheat, rye, or barley between five and seven months of age.

## How will I recognize a reaction?

### During an allergic reaction, your baby may have:

- A rash around the mouth, nose, and eyes
- Swelling of the lips, eyes, and face.
- An itchy mouth and throat; the throat may be swollen
- A runny or blocked nose and watery eyes
- Sickness and diarrhea

### Symptoms of a food intolerance include:

- Diarrhea or constipation, or blood or mucus in your baby's stools
- Colic
- Eczema
- Reflux

## How do I respond?

If you suspect your baby has had a reaction to a food, it is very important to seek professional advice and not simply withdraw the food from your baby's diet indefinitely, as your baby could miss out on vital nutrients. Make a note of what your baby ate and the symptoms, then avoid giving the food again until you've spoken to your pediatrician. Avoid, too, giving your baby similar foods to the one you suspect she reacted against. So if you think she reacted to cow's milk used in cooking, avoid other dairy products until you get advice. Depending on the severity of the reaction your pediatrician may refer your baby to an allergist for further investigation.

## Common culprits

The foods that most commonly cause allergic reactions are:

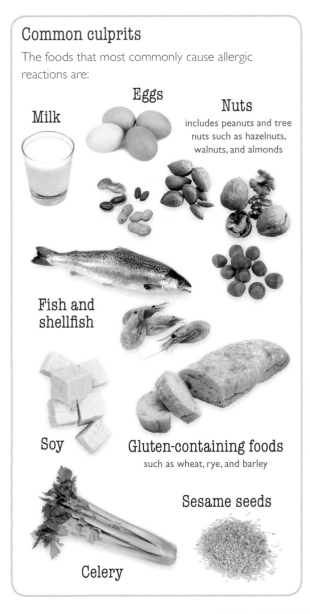

**Milk**

**Eggs**

**Nuts**
includes peanuts and tree nuts such as hazelnuts, walnuts, and almonds

**Fish and shellfish**

**Soy**

**Gluten-containing foods**
such as wheat, rye, and barley

**Sesame seeds**

**Celery**

# Reducing the risks

There's conflicting evidence about whether it's best to delay introducing allergenic foods or introduce them early in the weaning process. Current advice is that potentially allergenic foods can be safely introduced once your baby is six months old. Foods should be introduced one at a time (especially before six months) in order to quickly identify a potential allergy.

Some families are genetically more predisposed to food allergies. If a close member of your baby's family has severe eczema, asthma, hayfever, or allergies, she is at greater risk of developing an allergy than a baby whose family doesn't suffer. Also, if your baby has severe eczema, particularly if this started before three months, she has a higher risk of milk allergy. If her risk is higher, talk to your pediatrician about introducing allergenic foods. Breastfeeding while weaning may offer some protection against developing allergies, so if your baby has a family history, you may be able to reduce her risk by continuing to breastfeed while weaning.

# Living with an allergy

If your baby is diagnosed with an allergy, you will need to avoid the food as well as manufactured foods that could have traces of ingredients. These should be listed; the allergist can advise you on what names to look out for. A pediatric dietician can advise you on how to ensure your baby doesn't miss out on important nutrients.

When visiting others, let them know in advance that your baby can't have certain products, and bring along your own food in case they forget.

---

### A severe reaction (anaphylaxis) needing immediate medical attention includes:

- Wheezing, a cough, and breathing difficulties similar to an asthma attack
- Itchy skin or a red rash
- Swollen throat and tongue, which may affect voice
- A drop in blood pressure
- Confusion, dizziness, collapse, and unconsciousness
- If you suspect your baby has anaphylaxis, call 911 immediately for an ambulance.

# Weaning your *premature* baby

**If your baby was born early (before 37 weeks),** she may have missed out on some of the nutritional benefits of the last trimester of pregnancy, when babies build up stores of essential nutrients in the womb. In the first weeks and months, you may be advised to give your baby a special premie formula or supplements if she is breastfed to provide vitamins and minerals, including iron, to ensure she grows and develops well. When you start to wean your baby, you will want to ensure that her nutritional needs continue to be met.

## When should I wean my baby?

The actual date a premature baby is born on, rather than the expected due date you were given during pregnancy, is usually the date that is used to gauge when you should start to wean your baby onto solid foods. If your baby was very premature or very small at birth, then the medical team who cared for her in the first weeks and months should guide you on when to start weaning her onto solid foods. If your baby was only a few weeks premature and doesn't have any additional health problems, you will probably be advised to wean her around five to eight months from her actual birth date, and not to begin weaning before three months from her expected due date. As with all babies, she needs to show the signs that she is ready for solids (see p11). If you want further advice, talk to the medical team or your pediatrician.

## Will my baby take longer to wean?

Some premature babies develop conditions such as **reflux**. If this is the case, your pediatrician may give you advice on feeding or recommend a special formula or prescribe certain medications.

Premature babies do sometimes take a little longer to learn to eat than babies born closer to their due date. Also, if your baby has had complex medical issues, for example a cleft palate, you may need the support of specialist dietitians and speech therapists when you start to wean, which can affect how long weaning takes. The menu planners in this book are still ideal for your baby, just be guided by her development. For example, if she wants to eat, but is slow to use her hands, you may need to cook and mash or chop some of the vegetable finger foods into her meal and spoon feed for longer. She will catch up eventually, so try not to stress.

## Does my baby need more calories?

Each baby has their own individual nutritional requirements, whether or not they were premature. Pediatricians will assess your baby by weighing and measuring her: if she is steadily gaining weight as expected, they will be happy that she is receiving sufficient calories. Once you start weaning, the advice is the same as for all babies, and you will need to ensure that your baby doesn't stay on purées of pure vegetables or fruits for too long as these are low in calories. If your baby has any developmental problems, this can mean that you need to introduce new textures more slowly, in which case you may want to mix fruit and vegetable purées with your baby's usual milk, or add a little rice cereal to provide the calories your baby needs. If your baby had vitamin and mineral supplements after the birth, your health team will advise you on whether she needs to continue.

## Does my baby need bigger portion sizes?

It's important not to try to help a smaller baby catch up on growth by encouraging her to eat excessively. Unless a pediatrician has advised you otherwise, your baby needs to be weaned in the same way as other babies with the same portion sizes.

## Is my baby more susceptible to food allergies?

The digestive system of premature babies is not fully developed at birth, so it's natural to wonder if this means that your baby is at a greater risk than normal of developing food allergies. Reassuringly, several studies have shown that as long as you follow the guidelines for weaning and the advice of your pediatricians, this is not the case.

# Day-by-day
## planner

It's time to get started! In this section you'll find an introduction to each of the three stages of weaning, together with recipes for each age group and a menu plan for each day. The "menus" are no more complicated than one single taste at first, but the meals build up as the days and weeks go on.

# How to use the
## day-by-day planner

The day-by-day meal planners in this section cover the three stages of weaning: stage 1 up to seven months; stage 2 from seven to nine months, and stage 3 from nine to 12 months. The planners are designed to navigate you through each stage, providing a progression of textures and steadily introducing new tastes so that babies build up a repertoire of familiar foods and develop the ability to chew. The aim is that by the age of one, babies are eating foods from all the four main food groups and joining in with family meals.

## Making the planner work for you

Stage 1 can be adapted depending on the age at which you start to wean your baby. There are eight weeks of planners here, so if you start at five months, you can follow it to the letter if you wish. Page 41 has advice on how to speed up this stage if you start closer to six months. If you think your baby may be ready to start solids before five months, consult your pediatrician first; and never wean your baby before 17 weeks (see p11).

Each week provides a suggested daily menu for your baby appropriate for the weaning stage. So at the beginning of stage 1, there is just a single taste each day and by the end of this stage, your baby will be eating two simple meals a day. As your baby moves into stage 2, he will be having three regular meals each day. Each taste and meal is cross-referenced to the recipe pages. If you wish, you can follow the daily planners exactly, which will ensure that your baby receives a good balance of nutrients across the week. The quantities in most recipes make several meals, so you can freeze additional portions and use these when the recipe is repeated in a later week. From stage 2 onward, variations are provided each week if you'd prefer not to make what's on the planner, or if your baby has an allergy or intolerance to a certain food in the planner. And if you wish, you can simply use the planners as a reference tool, for inspiration and guidance on the balance of foods to aim for.

From stage 2 onward, there is a main meal each day and a lighter meal, as well as a breakfast suggestion. The main meal is usually listed as dinner, but this order doesn't need to be followed slavishly. If it's more convenient one day to have a main meal at lunchtime, then simply swap these around. Equally, many breakfast suggestions make good lunch options, or work well as desserts.

If you want to adapt the planner to suit the kind of day you're having, there are pages to help you. Pages 80–81 provide guidance on making the planner work when you're away from home, and pages 92–95 have other ideas for adapting the planners to suit your needs.

The planners are based on the more traditional route of weaning with purées. If you wish to follow baby-led weaning, you can still use the planners as a nutritional reference, providing you with ideas for different meals; if you wish, you can offer the same foods without puréeing.

If you are bringing up your baby as a vegetarian, you will find a good range of vegetarian recipes in the planners that you can use to form the basis of a varied diet for your baby. Many of these provide sources of protein in the form of dairy products or beans. Page 76 lists the main sources of protein in a vegetarian diet, so you will need to ensure that your baby's diet includes adequate amounts of these.

## Weaning twins

If you have twins, you may find that one baby is ready to wean earlier than the other, or that your twins progress at a different pace during the weaning process, perhaps one being happier to try new flavors, while the other is ready for lumps sooner. It's important to treat your twins as individuals and let each go at his own pace. You can adapt meals to suit each baby, perhaps removing a ground portion for one twin, then blending the rest of the meal for the other baby if he is not ready for this step up in texture. Batch cooking can also help you provide different tastes and textures for each one without having to cook up two different meals each time. As the aim of the weaning stages is for all babies to be joining in with family meals by 12 months, you should find that things even out as your twins get older.

## Thinking about allergies

With allergies on the rise in young children, there are certain foods that parents are currently advised to hold off on until after six months (see p41). The Stage 1 planners and recipes take this into account and avoid potentially allergenic foods under six months. (If you do start earlier than five months, make sure you avoid the foods listed on p41 until your baby reaches six months,

repeating the early weeks as necessary.) From stage 2 onward, recipes with peanuts are introduced. These usually appear as variations only in the planners so they're easy to avoid if you wish; the Vegetarian sauté (p126) appears in the main planner where peanuts appear as a variation to the main recipe, again making these easy to avoid. If you have a family history of allergies or feel unsure about introducing certain foods, talk to your doctor about the best approach.

## Dealing with choking

It's natural for parents to worry about their baby choking when they start to eat solid food. Gagging and choking are hazards as your baby learns to coordinate the muscles needed for chewing with breathing. It's common for babies to gag sometimes when they start on solids: this is a natural reflex that happens when there's a risk of choking. Your baby is learning to regulate the amount of food he has in his mouth and to coordinate chewing and swallowing, so it's natural that he struggles sometimes. Try not to panic if your baby gags, as usually he will manage to move the food to the front of his mouth. This is also a valuable lesson for him in the importance of chewing. Choking occurs when the airway becomes completely obstructed and your baby is unable to breathe. The first aid box on page 220 explains what to do if your baby chokes, but there is no substitute for attending a first-aid course or demonstration. Your local baby group may run one or check information online from first-aid societies such as The Red Cross.

You can reduce the risk of choking with simple measures such as removing skin on meats and fruits until your baby can chew more easily; halving foods such as grapes and cherry tomatoes that could block the windpipe if swallowed whole; and giving your baby lightly cooked foods before raw foods as he gets used to chewing. Always stay with your baby while he is eating so you can see if he is in trouble—a choking baby may not be able to cry or cough, so you can't rely on this to alert you.

# Introducing *Stage 1*

**This first phase of weaning, which usually starts at around five to six months** and continues to around seven months, introduces your baby to the idea that food isn't always liquid, and, if you are following the puréeing route, that food comes on a spoon, from which your baby has to learn to move the food from the front of her mouth to the back to swallow it.

## Progressing through the first stage

Your baby's first meals are mainly about experiencing new tastes and textures, as she will still be receiving everything she needs nutritionally from milk.

The menu planners and simple recipes guide you through the first weeks of weaning, suggesting ideal first foods for your baby, and ensuring that she learns to eat a wide range of nutritious foods. The planners for this stage cover a period of eight weeks, but can be extended or truncated if you wish to start earlier or later (see box, opposite).

## What your baby eats now

For the first few months of your baby's life, milk is the most important food in her diet, providing all the nutrients and calories she needs. She should continue her usual milk feeds when you introduce solids.

- At around six months, milk still plays a key role, but no longer provides all the iron and zinc your baby needs, so she needs solid foods now, too.

- Simple single flavors are the best first foods for your baby; these are usually vegetables, fruits, and cereals such as rice or millet. Giving your baby one food at a time allows her to identify the individual flavors. This can be especially important with some bitter vegetables that are essential to a healthy, nutritious diet. Your baby needs to learn what broccoli or spinach tastes like, so don't be tempted to add sweet fruit or parsnip to her first taste of greens.

- After some single flavors, blends can be introduced.

- Meat, poultry, fish, and beans which provide minerals such as iron and zinc, should be introduced from around six months.

## New experiences

Studies show that it can take up to 10 tries for new foods to be accepted by babies, and research shows that it is easiest to introduce new or difficult flavors before seven months of age, so it's important to offer your baby vegetables repeatedly early on in the weaning process. Once your baby has become used to these first flavors, meat, poultry, fish, and beans can be given toward the end of the first stage. Between five and seven months is a critical period when babies will accept difficult flavors such as green vegetables more readily than when these are left until after seven months.

Studies also show that babies who have only purées until nine months struggle to accept lumps. Make sure that early runny purées are followed up as soon as your baby can eat from a spoon with thicker ones, then mashed foods. Finger foods, whether given as part of a mixed diet alongside purées or alone if you are doing baby-led weaning (see p21) are crucial in helping your baby learn to chew and cope with lumps.

## STAGE 1—at a glance

**TEXTURE**

During the first stage of weaning, the texture of your baby's food should progress from **runny purées** to **thicker purées,** then **mashed food**.

**INTRODUCE**

By the end of stage 1, at around 7 months, your baby should have tried: fruits • vegetables • cereals, including wheat • first meats • fish • beans • dairy products

**AVOID**

Do not give processed meats such as sausages and ham, honey, liver, and whole nuts (see p19)

Runny purée

Thicker purée

Mashed food

---

## *Starting early or late*

If you start to give your baby first foods before she is six months old, you can move at a gentle pace through this first stage as milk will still be meeting her nutritional needs. We have given meal plans for eight weeks. If you introduce solids when your baby is five months old, you can follow the planner to the letter if you wish. If you want to provide a bit more variety, you can try some of the other first tastes and blends recipes from the recipe pages.

If you wean your baby before six months, the common advice is to avoid giving her eggs, liver, nuts and seeds, fish and shellfish, dairy products, gluten-containing products such as wheat, and citrus fruits. The planner has been designed so your baby doesn't encounter these foods until after six months.

If you've waited until the recommended six months, your baby's need for nutrients and calories has increased, so it's important to progress through this stage quickly as fruit and vegetable purées are low in calories as well as iron and zinc. By six months of age, your baby shouldn't stay on vegetable and fruit purées alone for more than a week or two before moving quickly onto meat, poultry, fish, and beans. This may mean not repeating some single flavors so often, especially fruits, which she is likely to favor anyway. The recipes often have common ingredients, so for example broccoli appears alone, then in combination with rice, then with rice and chicken, so if you wait until six months to wean, you could move from the simplest to more complex meals relatively quickly.

# Your baby's *first meal*

**Your baby's first meal can be quite an event** as you decide which food you are going to start with, when is the best time to give it, and worry about whether or not your baby will like it. Your baby will pick up on your emotions, whether you are anxious or excited as his first mouthful approaches, and will be aware of how you react when that food goes in, and perhaps comes out again. So it's important to try to be as relaxed and positive as possible, which will be most likely if you're well prepared.

## The first mouthful

Your baby's food is cooked and cooled and you're happy that it's the right consistency—a runny texture for first purées—so it's time to serve it up. Use the checklist here to help feeds go smoothly.

• Get your baby seated comfortably and securely in his high chair. If you are weaning before six months, your baby may not be able to sit upright easily in a high chair. You can hold him securely on your lap, or strap him into his bouncy chair if he has one.

• Put a bib on him—early feeding is messy, so this cuts down on endless changes of outfit.

• Use a soft-edged weaning spoon. If your baby is under six months old, this needs to be sterilized before use.

• Check that the food is the right temperature before giving it to your baby. Test a little on the inside of your wrist—it should be neither hot nor cold.

**1** Bring the spoon to your baby's lips and let him open his mouth.

**2** Gently move the spoon into his mouth so he can taste the food, letting him close his mouth around the spoon.

**3** Some food may come out! Scoop it up and pop it back in.

If he likes it, try another spoon. If he's resistant, don't force it. Wait and try again with the next meal.

> *Your baby's expression may not be quite what you expected. Wrinkling his nose doesn't necessarily mean he doesn't like a food. Try again and if he opens his mouth, you will know he is willing to give it a go. If he doesn't, just try another time.*

## Perfect timing

If you're feeling anxious about getting the timing right for your baby's first meal, bear in mind that he will be most responsive if he isn't too tired or too hungry. Your baby is used to satisfying his hunger quickly through drinking milk, so if he is very hungry, he won't cope well with the new experience of food on a spoon or tackling a finger food. Pick a time when he is alert and has had a small milk feed. Also choose a time that fits in with your day, too, as you need to be feeling calm and unrushed: it doesn't really matter whether this is breakfast time, lunchtime, or during the afternoon. Avoid later on in the day as you and your baby are more likely to be tired, and if he is unfortunate enough to react adversely to a food, you may miss any symptoms if you have put him to bed soon after eating the food.

## Good first purées

Your baby's first purées introduce him to a range of different vegetables, cereals, and fruits.

### First breakfast cereals

Rice is often the first food given, and rice cereal is fortified with vitamins and minerals. You can also try infant millet cereal.

A six-month-old baby can have cereals that contain grains such as wheat and barley, but look out for ones that are laden with sugar and/or salt.

### First vegetables

Green and cruciferous vegetables are important in the diet as they contain iron and other essential nutrients.

broccoli • spinach • cauliflower • kale

Root vegetables often taste sweet, and orange roots provide vitamin A. Potatoes, sweet potatoes, and yams are good sources of energy and useful for thickening purées.

carrot • parsnip • butternut squash • rutabaga • turnip • pumpkin • sweet potato • yam • potato

Other vegetables, which provide a mix of nutrients and tend to be liked by babies include:

peas • corn

### First fruits

Different colored fruits provide a range of vitamins and phytonutrients: naturally occurring substances that help protect the body from disease.

apple • pear • banana • apricot • avocado • mango • peach • blueberry

# How much is *enough?*

**Now that your baby is starting to eat solid food,** you may be concerned about just how much food he needs. In fact, he has a built-in mechanism to help him know when he is full—you simply need to learn to read the signs that he has had enough. As a rough guide, in the first few days he will probably only have a few mouthfuls, the equivalent of a teaspoon or two, at a time. The quantity will increase as he learns how to swallow food and starts to enjoy different flavors, building up to two or more tablespoons per meal as your baby moves into the second stage of weaning (see p76).

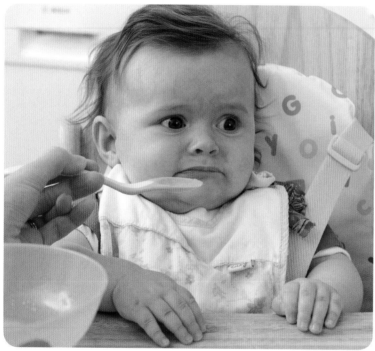

Read your baby's cues. If that final mouthful is refused, she's telling you she's full.

## Reading the signs

There are several signs to look out for to help you recognize when your baby has eaten enough:

- She may turn her head to one side to avoid another spoonful.
- She may refuse to open her mouth after she has eaten a few mouthfuls.
- She may spit food out. In the early stages, she may do this anyway if she hasn't lost her extrusion reflex, which causes her to push food to the front of her mouth. If this is the case, she may not be ready to wean and you might need to wait another week or two before trying again until she is able to move the food from the front to the back of her mouth.

### *Following your baby's lead*

Researchers have been looking at how to prevent young children from becoming overweight. Studies suggest that encouraging a baby to have more than she naturally eats or coercing her to clear her plate can have an adverse affect on her ability to self-regulate her intake of food. However, other research shows that being too concerned about overfeeding and restricting your child's intake of food is not helpful either. It can be tricky for parents to find the right balance. Try to be guided by your baby, watching for cues that she is full (see above) and not pressuring her to eat more if she seems reluctant.

## Your baby's milk feeds

Toward the end of stage one, your baby will be having two meals a day, including breakfast. However, these will consist of just a few spoonfuls of purée or cereal, so she will still be having her usual quantity of milk, around four to five breastfeeds, or approximately 20oz (600ml) formula each day.

As your baby moves through the weaning process, the quantity of milk will drop off gradually. If you continue breastfeeding, your baby will usually naturally reduce the amount of milk she takes, allowing your breasts to adjust and in turn reduce the amount of milk they produce. If you wish to wean your baby off the breast and onto formula, you will need to plan this more carefully. The advice is to do this slowly, if possible. This is more reassuring for your baby; she is used to the comfort of breastfeeding and is likely to become distressed if this is removed too quickly. Moving gradually from breast to bottle also reduces the risk of your breasts becoming uncomfortably engorged. Ideally, do this over a period of weeks, replacing one breastfeed a week with a bottle feed.

Your baby's enthusiasm for her food will be evident. Go at her pace, taking it slowly if she's a bit more cautious.

## Portion sizes

The portions shown below are suitable for babies who have accepted first tastes.
All babies vary in the amount they eat, and as they grow more is eaten at each meal.

| FOOD GROUP | TYPICAL MEAL | TYPICAL AMOUNT FOR UP TO 7 MONTHS OLD |
|---|---|---|
| Vegetables and fruits given singly | First tastes—any meal | 5 teaspoons per meal |
| Infant cereal or potato mixed with milk | Breakfast | 1–5 teaspoons of cereal/potato mixed with 4–10 teaspoons milk |
| Meat, poultry, fish, or beans mixed with vegetables | Lunch or dinner | 5 teaspoons per meal |
| Milk—formula or breastmilk | Throughout the day | Minimum 20oz (600ml) formula or 4–5 breastfeeds |
| Dairy foods alone or mixed with fruit | Dessert or breakfast | 5 teaspoons per meal |
| High fat/high sugar foods | Not suitable | Not suitable |

# Your *thirsty* baby

**Throughout the first year, your baby will continue to rely on breastmilk or formula** as a major source of energy and some nutrients. However, as she grows she will also need additional fluids for growth and to replace fluids lost in urine, stool, and sweating. Water is readily absorbed and used by the body and, other than milk, is the best drink for babies. Tap water is preferable as some mineral waters contain too much sodium or sulphate. Because she can't express her need for fluids, you will need to offer drinks with meals in addition to her daily milk.

## How much should my baby drink?

Before six months of age, bottlefed babies often need additional water to avoid constipation, while exclusively breastfed babies don't need extra water. Tap water is best, and under six months, you may want to boil and cool it before giving it to your baby. Once you introduce solids, your baby's need for water increases, whether she's breast or bottlefed. A baby between six and 12 months of age needs to drink around 34oz (1 liter) of fluid a day, which will be supplied in part by breastmilk or formula, and the balance from other drinks and foods. There's no need to boil and cool water first after six months. You don't need to measure out water for your baby in addition to her milk, but offer her a drink with her meals so that she can self-regulate the amount she needs. If she is unwell, she may need additional fluids, especially if she goes off her milk feeds.

It's important for your baby to learn how to control her appetite and to recognize the difference between hunger and thirst. If you give her too many drinks, with the exception of water, between meals, she may struggle to learn these innate cues.

### Cups and bottles

Once your baby is getting used to eating solids, it's time to ditch bottles and nipples and introduce lidded cups with spouts. This is because she needs to learn to sip rather than suck, and fluids, especially if they are sweetened, need to be in the mouth for as short a time as possible to minimize the risk of damage to her emerging teeth. You can buy fast-flow spouts for bottles to start your baby with at six months, but, as soon as possible, and certainly by 12 months, she should be drinking all bottled drinks, including formula, from a cup with or without a lid.

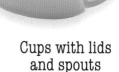

### Cups with lids and spouts

Cups with lids, spouts, and easy-to-hold handles are ideal first cups for your baby, helping to ease the transition from bottle to cup. Cups with spouts that flip up are easy flow, and non-spill when the spout is down; non-flip spouts require more sucking.

## What about juice and flavored drinks?

Even unsweetened fruit juices contain naturally present sugars, which is why milk and water are the best drinks for your baby. There are three main reasons to avoid sweetened drinks:

- Sweetened fluids can damage your baby's teeth.
- Your baby may develop a preference for sweetened foods and drinks.
- It is easy to over-consume sweetened drinks and this can lead to your baby being overweight.

If you are bringing up your baby as a vegetarian, you can offer her unsweetened fruit juice, diluted one part juice to 10 parts water, at mealtimes, as the vitamin C in the juice helps iron absorption from plant-based foods. Otherwise it's best to offer plain water at meal times.

If you do want to give your baby fruit juice, make sure it is unsweetened, diluted, and offer it only at mealtimes in a sippy cup, not a bottle with a nipple, so it can be quickly sipped. Don't give your baby drinks other than milk or water between meals. Any other drinks should definitely be avoided. Flavored milks are high in sugar, and soft drinks aren't suitable for babies or young children as they are acidic and damage teeth. Sweetened herbal drinks aren't suitable for babies, and don't be tempted to give even diluted tea or coffee as these contain caffeine and tannin, which interfere with iron absorption.

## Your baby's milk

If you've been breastfeeding and want to move to formula, which type is best for your baby? And if your baby has been on formula, should you change to a different type as he grows?

- Infant formula is suitable for babies up to and beyond one year.
- Growing-up milk is an enriched formula only suitable after one year, but talk to your pediatrician to determine if it is necessary for your child.
- Soy formula should only be used on the advice of a health professional, as this can be allergenic, and there are health concerns about the phyto-estrogens (plant hormones) it contains. Soy formula also contains sugars that can damage teeth.

## Other milks:

- Cow's milk isn't suitable as a drink until one year. At 12 months, whole cow's milk can be introduced as a drink, although the AAP recommends introducing low-fat milk at 12 months for children who have a family history of obesity or are overweight themselves. Low-fat milk can be introduced from two years of age if your toddler is growing well and has a healthy and varied diet.
- Soy milk is not suitable for children under the age of two as it is too low in iron, fat, and calories. Occasionally, a toddler may be advised to use a special toddler soy milk on medical grounds.
- Rice or nut milks aren't suitable for children under the age of five as they are nutritionally inadequate.

### Open cup with handles

By one year, possibly earlier, encourage your baby to drink from a cup without a lid.

### Open cup

As your child grows and her dexterity increases, she will manage a confident hold on a plastic cup without handles.

# Setting up *good habits*

**Your baby probably developed his taste buds before you even knew you were pregnant**, and they matured about 15 weeks after conception, just before the development of his taste receptors. Babies in the womb swallow amniotic fluid constantly, so by the time your baby was born, he would have experienced plenty of flavors from the foods you ate while you were pregnant.

## Shaping your baby's tastes

Your baby learns from watching you, and he will mimic your behavior, whether you like it or not! So he is much more likely to learn to love eating vegetables if he sees you and your partner eating and enjoying them. If, on the other hand, he senses that broccoli is a necessary evil that he is forced to eat but you won't countenance, you will have some difficulties ahead.

How does this feel?

Eating together is much more fun for your baby than eating alone, so whenever you can, eat with him. If possible, let him watch you prepare his meal, showing him what it contains. It is good for him to learn, for example, what a carrot looks like, so as he progresses from purées to mashed then chopped carrots, he is not surprised when it appears in a different form. Baby food is, after all, real food provided in an appropriate texture.

Toward the end of the first stage, you can start to introduce your baby to a range of soft finger foods, or you may start him off on finger foods at six months if you choose to follow baby-led weaning. Encouraging your baby to move toward more independent eating helps him to embrace new foods as he learns to eat on his own terms. Likewise, if your baby grabs the spoon while you feed him, let him have a go himself. If you're worried that not much of the food is making it to his mouth, you could use two spoons, one for him to hold and one that you keep to pop some food into his mouth between his attempts. Try not to get frustrated if this slows down mealtimes a little; letting him have a go helps him feel involved and interested in his food, so by the time he reaches his first birthday, he should be happy and relaxed joining in with family meals.

How does this taste?

## My baby won't eat!

It's not uncommon for babies to refuse food when they had previously been feeding well, or to resist the transition to solids. There are many reasons why babies refuse food; understanding why can help you avoid worrying about your baby's well-being.

- Your baby may not feel like eating if he's unwell, especially if it's early on in the weaning process when he will be comforted by the familiarity of milk rather than the newness of solids. Teething babies can also refuse food if their gums hurt and

they feel out of sorts. Try not to worry; simply try food again once he's feeling better, maybe starting with one of the foods that he clearly likes first.

- If your baby resists a food when first introduced, check that he is developmentally ready for solids (see p11). If he doesn't show these signs, you might need to hold off on solids for a while longer.
- Your baby may not feel like eating if he is already full on milk. Be guided by his appetite, and don't encourage him to finish bottles if he's unwilling.

# Made with love

You may have spent a lot of time preparing your baby's food. If this doesn't always get eaten—perhaps your baby isn't keen on a flavor or isn't very hungry—you may question whether it's worth the effort. So what are the advantages of homemade food, and are there times when commercial foods are fine for your baby?

## Pros of homemade food

- It's important for your baby to accept new textures. Homemade food has more variations in texture, and even the same dish won't be the same each time, so your baby learns it's okay when a dish feels different.

- Your baby will have experienced some flavors while in the womb and breastfeeding, so he's likely to be receptive to these when he encounters them again.

- If properly prepared and cooked, homemade food can contain more vitamin C and B group vitamins than pouches or jars of foods.

- Your baby can see foods being made so is less likely to be wary of ingredients.

- Homemade food is more cost effective, especially if making in bulk for freezing.

## Pros of commercial baby foods

- If the family diet is poor, using some commercial foods ensures some good nutrients for your baby.

- Strictly regulated sourcing means ingredients are sometimes better than ones used at home.

- Pouches and jars are convenient for traveling and as emergency pantry food.

- If parents have dietary restrictions, bought baby food can provide foods they can't eat.

- Some family foods, such as those containing salt, aren't suitable for babies.

# day-by-day meal planner Week 1

If you've waited until six months to begin weaning, you can skip week one, moving straight to week two with two tastes each day.

## Day 1
First taste
**Rice cereal** p58

## Day 7
First taste
**Pear** p59

## Day 2
First taste
**Carrot** p58

## Day 6
First taste
**Pear** p59

### *How much milk?*
Your baby needs to continue breastfeeding or having the same amount of infant formula each day.

## Day 3
First taste
**Carrot** p58

## Day 5
First taste
**Broccoli** p58

## Day 4
First taste
**Broccoli** p58

You don't need to follow the plan strictly, but do try to introduce broccoli, cauliflower, and spinach in the first two weeks.

# day-by-day meal planner
## Week 2

### Day 1
First taste
**Butternut squash** p59

Second taste
**Pear** p59

### Day 2
First taste
**Butternut squash** p59

Second taste
**Mango** p59

### Day 3
First taste
**Apple** p59

Second taste
**Broccoli** p58

### Day 4
First taste
**Spinach** p59

Second taste
**Apple** p59

### Day 5
First taste
**Spinach** p59

Second taste
**Banana** p59

### Day 6
First taste
**Cauliflower** p60

Second taste
**Mango** p59

### Day 7
First taste
**Cauliflower** p60

Second taste
**Blueberry** p60

### How much milk?
Your baby needs to continue breastfeeding or having the same amount of infant formula each day.

# day-by-day meal planner
## Week 3

If you've waited until six months to begin weaning, move onto blends and firmer textures quickly, minimizing the number of blends you use, and moving quickly onto meals. Or skip weeks one, three, and seven.

## Day 1
Breakfast
**Banana** p59

Second meal
**Pea** p60

## Day 2
Breakfast
**Apricot** p60

Second meal
**Pea** p60

## Day 3
Breakfast
**Apple** p59

Second meal
**Carrot and squash** p63

## Day 4
Breakfast
**Apple and plum** p63

Second meal
**Carrot and squash** p63

## Day 5
Breakfast
**Mango** p59

Second meal
**Cauliflower and sweet potato** p63

## Day 6
Breakfast
**Avocado** p61

Second meal
**Cauliflower and sweet potato** p63

## Day 7
Breakfast
**Millet and banana oatmeal** p68

Second meal
**Broccoli, pea, and potato** p65

### How much milk?
Your baby needs to continue breastfeeding or having the same amount of infant formula each day.

# day-by-day meal planner
## Week

4 3 2 1

### Day 1
Breakfast
Mango p59

Second meal
Zucchini, spinach,
and tomato p64

### Day 7
Breakfast
Apricot oatmeal p68

Second meal
Broccoli, pea,
and potato p65

### Day 2
Breakfast
Apple and yogurt p67

Second meal
Zucchini, spinach,
and tomato p64

### Day 6
Breakfast
Apple and yogurt p67

Second meal
Broccoli, pea,
and potato p65

### *How much milk?*
Your baby needs to continue
breastfeeding or having the
same amount of infant
formula each day.

### Day 3
Breakfast
Peach p61 or pear p59

Second meal
Carrot, leek,
and potato p64

### Day 5
Breakfast
Mango p59 or pear p59

Second meal
Parsnip and
sweet potato p65

### Day 4
Breakfast
Yogurt wih cinnamon
and pear p67

Second meal
Carrot, leek,
and potato p64

# day-by-day meal planner
## Week

5 4 3

Don't forget to offer your baby water with her meals (see p46).

### Day 1
Breakfast
Apricot and pear p66

Second meal
Corn, squash, and tomato p65

### Day 2
Breakfast
Banana oatmeal p68

Second meal
Beef, carrot, and potato p74

### Day 3
Breakfast
Teething biscuit with milk p70

Second meal
Corn, squash, and tomato p65

### Day 4
Breakfast
Apple and yogurt p67

Second meal
Beef, carrot, and potato p74

### Day 5
Breakfast
Banana slices and yogurt p67

Second meal
Cauliflower, cheese, and potato p71

### Day 6
Breakfast
Plum and yogurt p67

Second meal
Cauliflower, cheese, and potato p71

### Day 7
Breakfast
Apricot oatmeal p68

Second meal
Salmon and sweet potato p72

### How much milk?
Your baby needs to continue breastfeeding or having the same amount of infant formula each day.

# day-by-day meal planner
## Week 6

### Day 1
Breakfast
Orchard fruit
breakfast p70

Second meal
Salmon and
sweet potato p72

### Day 7
Breakfast
Apple and yogurt p67

Second meal
Butterbean and
sweet potato p73

### Day 2
Breakfast
Blueberry
and yogurt p67

Second meal
Lamb and apricots p75

### Day 6
Breakfast
Orchard fruits
breakfast p70

Second meal
Avocado and banana p66

*How*
*much milk?*

You may notice your baby
wants a little less of her milk
feed, but continue as you
have been doing.

### Day 3
Breakfast
Apricot and pear,
buttered toast p69

Second meal
Lamb and apricots p75

### Day 5
Breakfast
Teething biscuit
and milk p70

Second meal
Potato, spinach,
and ricotta p71

### Day 4
Breakfast
Mango and yogurt p67

Second meal
Potato, spinach,
and ricotta p71

# day-by-day meal planner
## Week 7

If you've waited until six months to begin weaning, you can skip weeks one, three, and seven.

### Day 1
Breakfast
Yogurt with cinnamon and pear p67

Second meal
Lentil, tomato, and coriander dhal p73

Soft pear slices

### Day 2
Breakfast
Apricot oatmeal p68

Second meal
Lentil, tomato, and coriander dhal p73

Plum and apple p63

### Day 7
Breakfast
Orchard fruits breakfast and toast fingers p70

Second meal
Chicken and Broccoli p74

Apricot and yogurt p67

### Day 3
Breakfast
Plum and yogurt p67

Second meal
Potato, spinach, and ricotta p71

Banana slices

### Day 6
Breakfast
Teething biscuit with milk and banana slices p70

Second meal
Cod, pea, and potato p72

Plum and apple p63

*How much milk?*

You may notice your baby wants a little less of her milk feed, but continue as you have been doing.

### Day 5
Breakfast
Banana and oat or millet oatmeal p68

Second meal
Cod, pea, and potato p72

Greek yogurt with apricot purée p70

### Day 4
Breakfast
Yogurt, banana slices, and buttered toast fingers p69

Second meal
Lamb and apricot p75

Blueberry purée with rice

# day-by-day meal planner
## Week

8 7 6 5 4 3

### Day 1
Breakfast
Hard-boiled egg p69

Second meal
Chicken and broccoli p74

Banana slices or purée

### Day 7
Breakfast
Hard-boiled egg and buttered toast p69

Second meal
Butterbean and sweet potato p73

Banana and pear slices

### Day 2
Breakfast
Greek yogurt with blueberry purée p70

Second meal
Salmon and sweet potato p72

Apple and mango or soft fruit pieces

### Day 6
Breakfast
Teething biscuit with milk and soft pear or mango pieces p70

Second meal
Butterbean and sweet potato p73

Blueberry purée with yogurt p67

### *How much milk?*
You may notice your baby wants a little less of her milk feed, but continue as you have been doing.

### Day 3
Breakfast
Sliced banana and yogurt p67

Second meal
Salmon and sweet potato p72

Greek yogurt with apricot purée p70

### Day 5
Breakfast
Apricot oatmeal and buttered toast p69

Second meal
Beef, carrot, and potato p74

Peach slices with yogurt p67

### Day 4
Breakfast
Yogurt with cinnamon and pear p67

Second meal
Beef, carrot, and potato p74

Apple purée p59

# Single *tastes*

**The first tastes your baby tries** give him the chance to try small amounts of different foods and learn that food comes in forms other than liquid. There are plenty of purées here to try over the first couple of weeks. Some, such as banana, avocado, or rice cereal are made up fresh each time, while others can be made in batches to freeze. Starting off with single flavors helps your baby distinguish different foods. Try to give vegetables more often than fruit in the first week or two so your baby doesn't develop a taste for sweet foods. As your baby gets used to solids, thicken purées by using less water or milk, or by adding a little rice cereal or mashed potato. The portion sizes here are suitable for stage 1 weaning (see pp44–45).

## *Freezing your baby's food*

It's best to cook foods before freezing them. Where a purée or meal is suitable for freezing, after cooking remove a portion to eat immediately, then cool the remainder before freezing in a container (see p27) marked with the date and food. Use all purées within six months, defrosting them in a fridge at less than 39.2°F (4°C).

## Rice cereal

This easily dissolvable vitamin-fortified powder is a popular first food, letting your baby adjust to a new texture while enjoying the familiar flavor of milk. Rice cereal can also be used to thicken purées as your baby progresses through the first stage of weaning.

 1 portion

### ingredients
Your **baby's usual milk**
**Rice cereal**

### method
**1** Follow the instructions on the package: usually 1 teaspoon rice cereal is used for every tablespoon of milk.

## Carrot

Carrots are a wonderful source of vitamin A, and their sweet taste makes them a popular vegetable with babies and toddlers alike.

 7–8 mins  4–5 portions

### ingredients
1 large **carrot**
¼ cup cooled boiled **water**, or your **baby's usual milk**

### method
**1** Peel the carrot and trim off the top and bottom. Cut into ½in (1cm) cubes or slice thinly.

**2** Steam for 7–8 minutes, or until tender.

**3** Cool slightly, then purée with the water or milk.

## Broccoli

This is high in vitamins A and C and also provides some iron; it's worth introducing this purée early as broccoli is an important staple of a healthy diet.

 8–10 mins

 8–10 portions

### ingredients
5½oz (150g) **broccoli florets**, washed
½ cup cooled boiled **water**, or your **baby's usual milk**

### method
**1** Steam the broccoli for 8–10 minutes until tender.

**2** Cool slightly, then purée with the water or milk.

## Pear

Pears are a classic first weaning food as they don't cause allergic reactions. Use ripe pears that are not too grainy, such as Bartlett or D'anjou.

  5–6 mins

8–10 portions ❄

### ingredients

2 medium ripe **pears**
cooled boiled **water**, or your
   **baby's usual milk**, if required

### method

**1** Peel the pears, quarter, and remove the cores. Dice and steam for 5–6 minutes.

**2** Cool slightly, then purée the pears with the water or milk if required.

## Squash

Butternut or other squashes such as pumpkin or acorn squash purée easily and have protective vitamin A. Use pre-cut fresh or frozen squash if you want a small quantity.

    10–12 mins

6–8 portions ❄

### ingredients

5½oz (150g) **butternut squash**
⅓ cup cooled boiled **water**, or your
   **baby's usual milk**

### method

**1** Peel the squash and cut into cubes, around ½–¾in (1–2cm) in size.

**2** Steam for 10–12 minutes or until tender.

**3** Cool slightly; purée with water or milk.

## Mango

Rich in vitamin C, mangoes make a tasty purée. The fruit should yield slightly when pressed. Use unsweetened canned mango purée when fresh is out of season.

  2 portions

### ingredients

3–3½oz (80–100g) or about one quarter fresh ripe **mango**, cut into cubes

### method

**1** Purée the mango cubes until smooth.

**2** Use half immediately, then refrigerate the rest in an airtight container for 24 hours.

★ *Variation: Mix with strawberry purée and/or yogurt for a simple and delicious dessert or breakfast.*

## Apple

Universally enjoyed, this is often a first fruit a baby eats. Any apple will do, but a sweet, softer flesh purées more easily than a crisp apple.

  7–9 mins

6–8 portions ❄

### ingredients

2 medium **apples**
⅓ cup cooled boiled **water**
   or your **baby's usual milk**

### method

**1** Peel and core the apples. Cut into quarters, then cut each quarter into smaller pieces, about ½ (1cm) in size.

**2** Steam for 7–9 minutes until soft. Remove from the heat.

**3** Cool slightly then purée the apple with the water or milk.

## Spinach

Providing vitamins A, C, and K, and iron, spinach has great nutritional credentials. You can add some of your baby's milk to sweeten it a little.

  5–6 mins

6–7 portions ❄

### ingredients

5½oz (150g) fresh **spinach leaves**
2 tbsp cooled boiled **water** or
   your **baby's usual milk**, if needed

### method

**1** Wash the leaves. Drain in a colander, then place in a large lidded pan.

**2** Bring to a boil, then simmer and cook until the leaves wilt.

**3** Cool slightly, then purée, adding water or milk, if required.

★ *Tip: Add to other foods once accepted.*

## Banana

Possibly an all-time baby favorite, banana makes a very easy purée. With no preparation or cooking required, all you need is a fork, plate, and banana for an instant meal on the go.

  1 portion

### ingredients

½ small ripe **banana**

### method

**1** Peel the banana and chop or slice roughly.

**2** Using a fork, mash until the banana becomes a smooth purée. Use immediately.

# Cauliflower

This is a good source of vitamin C and the B vitamin folate. Both nutrients are reduced during cooking, so steam and cool rapidly to preserve as many nutrients as possible.

 8–10 mins

 6–8 portions

### ingredients

5½oz (150g) **cauliflower** florets, washed

⅓ cup cooled boiled **water** or your **baby's usual milk**

### method

**1** Steam the cauliflower florets for 8–10 minutes, or until tender.

**2** Cool slightly, then purée with the water or milk.

# Blueberry

Blueberries purée easily, but because of their seeds and skin, they don't become absolutely smooth, so you may want to wait to make this one until your baby has become accustomed to eating from a spoon. Add to yogurt or a little rice cereal to make a simple dessert or breakfast.

 5 mins  5–6 portions

### ingredients

3½oz (100g) **blueberries**
2 tbsp **water**

### method

**1** Wash the blueberries and place in a small saucepan with the water.

**2** Heat for 3–4 minutes, breaking up the berries with a wooden spoon.

**3** When the berries have softened, remove from the heat and cool slightly. Blend with the liquid until you have a purée.

★ **Variation:** *If you want a thicker purée, add 2 teaspoons of rice cereal, stirring well until it is mixed thoroughly.*

# Pea

Peas are sweet and full of vitamin C. However, they can be difficult to purée completely finely, so it's probably best to hold back on giving your baby this purée until first tastes are well established. Use frozen petit pois rather than garden peas as they are less fibrous and easier to purée.

 5–6 mins  4–6 portions

### ingredients

3½oz (100g) frozen **petit pois**

⅓ cup cooled boiled **water** or your **baby's usual milk**

### method

**1** Steam the peas for 5–6 minutes until very tender.

**2** Cool slightly, then purée with the water or milk.

# Apricot

Fresh apricots have only a short season, so at other times of the year make this popular favorite using dried apricots, or simply purée canned apricots in fruit juice. This purée is great to pop into some yogurt or cottage cheese for a simple breakfast or dessert.

 17–20 mins  8–10 portions

### ingredients

3½ oz (100g) dried **apricots**

1 cup **water**

### method

**1** Place the apricots in a small saucepan and pour in the water.

**2** Cover with a lid and bring to a boil, then reduce the heat and simmer until the apricots are soft.

**3** Cool slightly and purée with the cooking liquid until runny, adding more water if required.

# Avocado

These provide energy from healthy fats as well as vitamin E, and are an enjoyable creamy first food. All you need to prepare them is a sharp knife and a fork for mashing, making avocados an easily portable meal for babies. Lemon or lime juice prevents the flesh from browning, but isn't essential.

  1 portion

### ingredients

¼ ripe **avocado**

1 tsp **lemon** or **lime juice**, optional

### method

**1** Cut the avocado flesh into cubes and sprinkle with the juice, if using.

**2** Mash with a fork until you have a smooth, creamy purée, and use immediately.

*✱ Variation: Mix avocado and banana for a popular baby meal (see p66).*

# Peach

Seasonal peaches or nectarines make a runny purée, suitable from early on. Like most soft fruit, they are best fresh. As soon as your baby can hold foods, you can give pieces of peeled peach.

  1 portion

### ingredients

1 small or ½ medium ripe **peach** or **nectarine**

### method

**1** Using a sharp knife, remove the skin and pit the peach or nectarine (see tip, below).

**2** Cut the flesh into chunks, purée until smooth, and use immediately.

*✱ Tip: To remove the skin, fill a small bowl with boiling water and place the fruit in the bowl for 1 minute. Remove with a slotted spoon, and using a small sharp knife, peel away the skin.*

# Plum

These are a good source of vitamin A. Choose ripe fruit that yield a little when gently pressed.

 10–12 mins  5–6 portions

### ingredients

2 medium **plums**, washed and pitted, cut into quarters

½ cup **water**

### method

**1** Place the plums and water in a saucepan and bring to a boil.

**2** Reduce the heat, cover, and simmer until the fruit is tender.

**3** Cool slightly before puréeing.

# Rutabaga

This is an inexpensive root vegetable that has a slight sweetness, making it popular with babies.

 7–8 mins  6–8 portions

### ingredients

5¾oz (160g) or one small piece of **rutabaga**, peeled and cut into

¼in (5mm) cubes
⅓ cup cooled boiled **water** or your **baby's usual milk**

### method

**1** Steam the rutabaga for 7–8 minutes or until tender.

**2** Cool slightly, then purée with the water or milk.

# Parsnip

With a mild, sweet flavor and creamy texture, parsnips are a favorite first vegetable, and this purée is ideal for adding to other vegetable, meat, or poultry purées in the early weeks of weaning. Choose smaller parsnips, as large ones tend to be a bit tough in the center so purée less well.

 5–6 mins  6–8 portions

### ingredients
1 medium or 2 small **parsnips**

⅛ cup cooled boiled **water**, or your **baby's usual milk**

### method
**1** Peel the parsnip and trim off the top and bottom. Slice thinly, discarding any particularly woody parts. Steam for 5–6 minutes or until tender.

**2** Cool slightly, then purée with the water or milk.

# Corn

Once your baby has become used to a few flavors and you are making less runny purées, try corn. Like peas, corn is more fibrous than some vegetables and the smoothness of your purée will depend on the efficiency of your processor or blender. Frozen corn can be used to make a simple, cost effective purée. Corn provides essential vitamin B3 (niacin).

 3–5 mins  4–6 portions

### ingredients
3½oz (100g) frozen **corn**

¼ cup cooled boiled **water**, or your **baby's usual milk**

### method
**1** Steam the corn for 3–5 minutes until tender.

**2** Cool slightly, then purée with the water or milk.

# Sweet potato

Unlike ordinary potatoes, sweet potatoes purée easily, making them a great baby food. They also provide generous amounts of vitamin A.

 10–12 mins  6–8 portions

### ingredients
5½oz (150g) or 1 small **sweet potato**

½ cup cooled boiled **water** or your **baby's usual milk**

### method
**1** Peel the sweet potato and cut into ½in (1cm) cubes. Steam for 10–12 minutes until soft.

**2** Cool slightly, then purée with the water or milk.

# Papaya

Papaya is rich in protective vitamin C. Just half a small ripe papaya will make a simple purée for your baby. This is best prepared and served fresh.

  1–2 portions

### ingredients
½ small ripe **papaya**

### method
**1** Remove and discard the black seeds from the fruit. Using a teaspoon, scoop out the pink flesh, discarding the skin.

**2** Mash the flesh to make a purée.

**3** Use immediately, then refrigerate any unused purée in an airtight container and use within 24 hours.

# First *blends*

**As your baby becomes used to a few single flavors**, you can start to combine purées to make different dishes, either by mixing ones you have already made and frozen, or by trying out some new recipes from this section. The more accustomed your baby becomes to eating from a spoon, the less runny the purée should be. Some of the recipes in this section include a tablespoon of vegetable oil. This ensures your baby is getting calories and monounsaturated fats in addition to vitamins and some minerals from vegetables. As with the single tastes, where suitable for freezing, cool any remaining purée and freeze with the date and name of the food (see p58).

# Carrot and pumpkin/ butternut squash

These autumn flavors are rich in vitamin A. Use frozen or prepared squash if you're not using the whole squash.

 8 mins    4 portions

### ingredients

2oz (60g) or 1 small **carrot**, peeled and cut into cubes
3½oz (100g) peeled **butternut squash** or **pumpkin**, cut into cubes
1 tbsp **vegetable oil**

### method

**1** Steam the vegetables until they are tender, about 8 minutes. Cool slightly, then purée with the oil until smooth, adding your baby's usual milk, if needed.

# Plum and apple

When plums are in season, this often forgotten fruit provides useful amounts of protective substances called polyphenols. Buy ripe plums that will be juicy and sweet.

 6–8 mins    5–6 portions

### ingredients

1 medium **apple**, peeled, cored, and roughly chopped
2 medium **plums**, washed, pitted, and quartered

### method

**1** Place all the ingredients with ½ cup water in a small lidded saucepan and bring to a boil.

**2** Stir, reduce the heat, and cover. Allow to simmer, stirring occasionally until the fruit is tender. Cool slightly, then purée.

# Cauliflower and sweet potato

With vitamin C and folate, cauliflower pairs up well with vitamin A-rich sweet potato.

 8–10 mins    4–5 portions

### ingredients

5½oz (150g) or 1 small **sweet potato**, peeled and diced
2½oz (70g) or 2 **cauliflower florets**
1 tbsp **vegetable oil**
3 tbsp **milk**

### method

**1** Steam the sweet potato and cauliflower until tender, around 8 minutes. Cool slightly, then blend with the oil and milk to make a thick purée.

# Carrot, leek, and potato

These simple flavors are enhanced by gently cooking the leek. The carrots are a cheap source of essential vitamin A.

 10–12 mins  5–6 portions

## ingredients

3in (8cm) piece of **leek**—preferably the white part
1 tbsp **vegetable oil**
3½oz (100g) **carrots**, peeled and thinly sliced
4oz (120g) **potatoes**, peeled and quartered
**milk**, if needed

## method

**1** Slice the leek into small circles. Heat the oil in a small saucepan and gently cook the leek until soft.

**2** Add the carrots and ½ cup water, stir, and cover. Simmer gently until the carrots are soft, adding 1–2 tablespoons more water if required.

**3** Meanwhile, steam the potatoes until tender. Press them through a ricer into a clean bowl, or use a potato masher.

**4** Purée the carrot and leek and stir into the mashed potato, adding a little milk if you need to adjust the texture.

# Zucchini, spinach, and tomato

As weaning progresses and there's more food to prepare, you won't want to spend more time than is necessary in the kitchen. Peeling and seeding tomatoes can be avoided by using a bottle or carton of long-life unsalted sieved tomato purée. This is heat-treated in its preparation so doesn't require further cooking, making it easy to add while puréeing. Tomatoes provide valuable vitamin C, which helps the body absorb iron.

 7–8 mins  5–6 portions

## ingredients

1 tbsp **vegetable oil**
3½oz (100g) **zucchini**, washed and cut into cubes
3½oz (100g) **spinach leaves**, rinsed
3–5 tbsp **tomato purée**
pinch of **ground nutmeg** (optional)

## method

**1** Heat the oil in a saucepan and cook the zucchini without browning until just soft.

**2** Add the spinach leaves, stir, and cover. Continue to cook over low heat for 3–4 minutes until the spinach has wilted, then remove from the heat.

**3** Purée the zucchini and spinach mixture and then stir in as much tomato purée as you need for an appropriate texture. Stir in the nutmeg if using.

**✱ Tip:** *You can stir in a little rice cereal to adjust the texture if the purée is too runny.*

# Broccoli, pea, and potato

Most babies enjoy potato and it makes the texture transition from runny purées to thicker foods easy. As potato doesn't purée well, use a potato ricer or masher, mixing in milk or oil before stirring in other vegetables.

 8–10 mins     5–6 portions    ❄

## ingredients

3½oz (100g) **potatoes**, peeled and quartered
3½ oz (100g) **broccoli florets**, washed
1¾oz (50g) frozen **peas**
1 tbsp **vegetable oil**
**milk**, if needed

## method

**1** Steam or boil the potatoes until tender.

**2** Meanwhile, steam the broccoli and peas together until tender.

**3** In a clean bowl, press the potatoes through a ricer, or use a potato masher if you prefer, and stir in the oil.

**4** Blend the peas and broccoli to make a purée, adding milk if necessary, and stir into the mashed potato.

# Parsnip and sweet potato

A sweet root vegetable combination, sweet potato is a fabulous source of vitamin A and provides essential vitamins E and C. Choose smaller parsnips as large ones tend to be a bit tough in the center.

 10–12 mins     6–8 portions

## ingredients

3½oz (100g) **parsnips**, peeled and cut into chunks
7oz (200g) **sweet potatoes**, peeled and cut into chunks
3–5 tbsp **milk**

## method

**1** Steam the parsnips and sweet potatoes together until they are both tender.

**2** Cool slightly, then purée with the milk to create a smooth consistency.

**★ Tip:** *This purée can be added to a mashed potato, or used to add to stews or soups, where it will help thicken the dish as well as provide essential nutrients.*

# Corn, squash, and tomato

This makes a lovely transition to a more textured purée, and is a good source of vitamins A, C, and B3 (niacin).

 12 mins     3–4 portions    ❄

## ingredients

2½oz (75g) **butternut squash**, peeled and diced
2½ oz (75g) frozen **corn**
¼ cup **tomato purée**
1 tbsp **vegetable oil**

## method

**1** Steam the squash for 10 minutes, then add the corn and cook until tender.

**2** Cool slightly, then blend with the tomato purée and oil to make a thick purée.

# Apricot and pear

This sweet fruity mix is a healthy treat for your baby, packed with vitamins C and E.

 17–20 mins  10 portions

## ingredients

3½oz (100g) dried **apricots**
2 medium ripe **pears**, peeled, cored, and diced
1 cup **water**

## method

**1** Place the dried apricots in a small saucepan and pour in the water. Cover and bring to a boil, then simmer until the apricots are soft. Cool slightly.

**2** Meanwhile, steam the pears for 5–6 minutes.

**3** Combine the ingredients together with the cooking liquid, then purée.

# Avocado and banana

This classic combination is a favorite with babies. Rich in vitamin E and healthy monounsaturated fat, avocado, like banana, is easily portable for a meal on the go.

  1 portion

## ingredients

¼ ripe **avocado**, sliced
¼ ripe **banana**, sliced

## method

**1** Mash the avocado and banana with a fork until you have a smooth purée.

**2** Use immediately.

# Broccoli, leek, and potato

As you build up your baby's repertoire of vegetables, try adding gently cooked scallions for flavor.

 8–10 mins  6–7 portions

## ingredients

1 tbsp **vegetable oil**
1¾oz (50g) **leeks**, washed and thinly sliced
5½oz (150g) **potatoes**, peeled and quartered

5½ oz (150g) **broccoli florets**, washed
**milk**, if needed

## method

**1** Heat the oil in a small saucepan and gently cook the leeks, for about 5 minutes, stirring often until softened but not browned. Remove from the heat.

**2** Meanwhile, steam or boil the potatoes until tender, about 5 minutes. Steam the broccoli until tender, then purée with the leeks, adding milk if needed.

**3** In a clean bowl, press the potatoes through a ricer, or use a potato masher, and mix with the leek and broccoli mixture.

# Breakfasts

You can introduce variety into your baby's breakfasts by combining fruit purées with cereals or yogurts. Whole-grain infant cereals provide an excellent source of iron and fiber and can be easily mixed together with baby's milk or water. For early weaning, you can make your own infant cereal with grains you have at home if you prefer; purée rolled oats into a fine flour in your food processor or blender. As your baby gets used to solids, you can try giving him unblended oats.

## Yogurt with cinnamon and pear

Pear purée mixes well with yogurt for a tasty first breakfast. Stirring in a pinch of cinnamon makes it just a little different for your baby.

  1 portion

### ingredients
2 tbsp full-fat **natural yogurt**
2 tsp **pear purée** (see p59)
pinch of **ground cinnamon**

### method
**1** Mix together the yogurt, pear, and cinnamon and serve immediately.

## Apple and yogurt breakfast

Yogurt is a good source of calcium and magnesium for your baby's bones and teeth. Full-fat natural yogurt mixed with a simple purée such as apple, pear, banana, or blueberry makes a nutritious start to the day.

1 portion

### ingredients
2 tbsp full-fat **natural yogurt**
2 tsp **apple purée** (see p59)

### method
**1** Mix together the yogurt and apple and serve immediately.

Apple and yogurt breakfast

# Apricot oatmeal

Oatmeal made with flaked oats may be too lumpy for your baby to start with, but you can easily make it into a finer grain by puréeing in the processor.

 2–3 mins  1 portion

## ingredients

1 tbsp infant **oatmeal**, or **rolled oats** for an older baby

⅓ cup **baby's usual milk**

1 tbsp **apricot purée** (see p60)

## method

**1** Place the oatmeal and milk in a small pan and heat, stirring constantly.

**2** When the mixture thickens, remove from the heat and cool to body temperature.

**3** Stir in the apricot purée and serve immediately.

*Apricot oatmeal*

# Banana oatmeal

Comforting nutritious oatmeal with a hint of banana is quick and easy to make and a lovely way for your baby to start the day.

 2–3 mins  1 portion

## ingredients

1 tbsp infant **oatmeal**, or **rolled oats** for an older baby

¼ cup **baby's usual milk**

few slices of **banana**

## method

**1** Place the oatmeal and milk in a small pan and heat, stirring constantly.

**2** When the mixture thickens, remove from the heat and cool to body temperature.

**3** Meanwhile, mash the banana with a fork until smooth and stir into the oatmeal.

*✻ Microwave version:* *Mix the oats and milk in a microwaveable bowl and cook on high heat for 30 seconds (800W oven). Stir and cook for another 10 seconds. (The timing will vary according to the power of your microwave.) Once thickened, remove from the microwave, stir, and let cool before adding the banana.*

# Millet and banana oatmeal

Millet is a gluten-free grain that makes a simple first breakfast, providing iron and vitamin B3. Infant millet cereal is perfect for this simple oatmeal.

 2–3 mins  1 portion

## ingredients

1 tbsp infant **millet cereal**

¼ cup **baby's usual milk**

few slices of **banana**

## method

**1** Place the millet and milk in a small pan and heat, stirring constantly.

**2** When the mixture thickens, remove from the heat and cool to body temperature.

**3** Meanwhile, mash the banana with a fork until smooth and stir into the oatmeal.

*✻ Tip: For a bigger appetite, simply double the ingredients.*

# Hard-boiled egg

Storing eggs in the fridge will keep them fresh. Make sure eggs are well cooked in the early stages of weaning.

 10 mins  1 portion

## ingredients

1 **egg**

## method

**1** Fill a small pan with enough water to cover an egg. Bring to a boil.

**2** Gently lower the egg into the pan, being careful not to crack its shell. Boil for around 10 minutes.

**3** Let cool, then remove the shell and slice the egg into quarters for your baby.

# Buttered toast

Once your baby is able to hold foods, she can enjoy some toast fingers. She may find white or whole wheat bread easier to eat at first than bread with cracked grains or seeds. Use a monounsaturated spread such as olive, or unsalted butter if you prefer, or try full-fat cream cheese. Your baby may like to dip her toast into a fruit purée.

 2 mins  1 portion ❄

## ingredients

½ slice **white** or **whole wheat** bread

**olive spread**, or **unsalted butter**

## method

**1** Toast the bread, then cut it into 2–3 sections to make toast fingers.

**2** Spread with the chosen topping.

Buttered toast

# Greek yogurt and fruit purée

Sweeten up Greek yogurt by adding one of the fruit purées you've made already. Your baby needs full-fat Greek yogurt to provide essential calories.

  1 portion

## ingredients

2 tbsp full-fat **Greek yogurt**

2 tsp **fruit purée** (see pp59–66)

## method

**1** Mix together the Greek yogurt and purée and serve immediately.

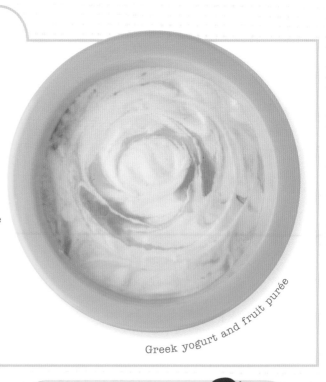

*Greek yogurt and fruit purée*

# Teething biscuit with milk

Teething biscuits are a popular first breakfast as they soak up milk easily and quickly become soft, making them simple for your baby to eat. Use either specially formulated baby teething biscuits, or standard ones.

  1 portion

## ingredients

½ **teething biscuit**
¼ cup of your **baby's**

**usual milk**, cold or warmed

## method

**1** Crumble the teething biscuit into a bowl and pour in the milk.

**2** Allow to soften for a couple of minutes and stir. Serve immediately.

# Orchard fruits breakfast

Vary your baby's breakfasts by adding different fruit purées to teething biscuits.

  1 portion

## ingredients

½ **teething biscuit**
¼ cup of your **baby's usual milk**, cold or

warmed
1 tbsp **plum and apple purée** (see p63)

## method

**1** Crumble the teething biscuit into a bowl and pour in the milk.

**2** Allow to soften for a couple of minutes, then stir in the plum and apple purée. Serve immediately.

**★ Tip:** *If you have frozen portions of fruit purée, pop one in a bowl and defrost in the microwave before you start. Or if you are very organized, defrost in the fridge the night before.*

# First *meals*

**When your baby has become used to eating food from a spoon** and accepts a range of different single and blended flavors, it's important to introduce more protein-rich foods such as meat, poultry, fish, beans, and cheese into her diet. Meat, fish, poultry, and beans all contain iron, essential for her growth and development (pp14–17). If you've waited until six months to start weaning, make sure you introduce these iron-rich purées within a couple of weeks. See page 27 for advice on freezing additional portions.

## Cauliflower, cheese, and potato

A good source of calcium and vitamin C, sauce-rich cauliflower and cheese is a family favorite.

 5 mins      10–15 mins

 5–6 portions

### ingredients

3½oz (100g) **potatoes**, peeled and cut into chunks
7oz (200g) **cauliflower florets**, washed

¼ cup **milk**
1½oz (40g) **Cheddar cheese**, grated

### method

**1** Steam the potatoes and cauliflower together until tender.

**2** Using tongs, remove the cauliflower and purée with the milk in a blender until smooth.

**3** Press the potatoes through a ricer into a clean bowl, or use a potato masher, and stir in the cheese.

**4** Mix together the potato and cauliflower mixtures. Cool slightly before serving.

## Potato, spinach, and ricotta

Ricotta is a mild soft cheese, which adds protein and calcium to this yummy mixture. You can add milk or water to adjust the texture if this is too firm.

 5 mins      5–6 portions      10–15 mins

### ingredients

7oz (200g) **potatoes**
1 tbsp **vegetable oil**
2 **scallions**, trimmed, washed, and cut into small pieces
3½oz (100g) **spinach leaves**, washed and drained
1¾oz (50g) **ricotta cheese**
pinch of grated **nutmeg** (optional)

### method

**1** Peel the potatoes, cut into chunks, and steam until soft, about 5 minutes.

**2** Meanwhile, heat the oil in a medium saucepan and gently cook the scallions until soft, without browning them.

**3** Add the spinach, cover, and cook for 3–4 minutes until the spinach has wilted.

**4** Press the cooked potato through a ricer or mash until soft and stir in the ricotta cheese.

**5** Purée the spinach and scallion mixture and stir into the cheesy potato along with a pinch of grated nutmeg if using. Cool slightly before serving.

**★ Variation:** *If you prefer, you can use ¾oz (20g) leeks instead of scallions.*

Salmon and sweet potato

# Salmon and sweet potato

Salmon is a popular oily fish, providing essential omega 3 fatty acids for your baby's eye and brain development. Mixed with sweet potato and carrots, this colorful meal is likely to become a favorite.

 5 mins    15–17 mins    6–8 portions

## ingredients

7oz (200g) **sweet potatoes,** peeled and cut into ½in (1cm) cubes

3½oz (100g) or 1 large **carrot,** peeled and cut into ½in (1cm) cubes

2½oz (75g) skinless **salmon fillet**

½ cup cooled and boiled **water** or **milk**

## method

**1** Place the sweet potato and carrot pieces in a steamer over a pan of boiling water and cook for 5 minutes.

**2** Run your finger over the fish to check for any bones. Remove any you find. Loosely wrap the fish in a piece of foil and place it on top of the vegetables. Continue steaming for 10–12 minutes.

**3** Remove the parcel of fish and check if it is cooked by inserting a knife to separate the flakes. The fish should look opaque and be the same color throughout. If it isn't, return to the pan and steam for a few minutes more.

**4** Check if the vegetables are tender and remove from the pan to cool slightly.

**5** Mix the salmon, sweet potato, and carrots in a blender with the water or milk to make a smooth purée.

✱ **Variation:** *Use a trout fillet instead of salmon.*

# Cod, pea, and potato

You can substitute the cod here for other responsibly sourced fish such as haddock, tilapia, halibut, or pollock. These white fish are simple to cook and easy for your baby to digest. Using peas adds sweetness and is a good step on the way to your baby enjoying fish pie with the rest of the family.

 5 mins     15–18 mins     7–10 portions

## ingredients

7oz (200g) **potatoes,** peeled and cut into ½–¾in (1–2 cm) cubes

3½oz (100g) skinless **cod fillet**

¼ tsp finely chopped **mint** (optional)

5½ oz (150g) frozen **petit pois**

¼ cup **milk,** plus more if needed

2 tsp **monounsaturate-rich spread** (such as olive)

## method

**1** Place the potatoes in a steamer and cook for 5 minutes, or until tender.

**2** Meanwhile, run your finger over the fish to check for any bones, removing any you find. Loosely wrap the fish in a piece of foil and sprinkle with the mint, if using.

**3** Place the peas in a separate steamer with the fish parcel over it, and steam for 6–7 minutes.

**4** Remove the fish parcel and the peas and check to see that the fish is cooked by inserting a knife to separate the flakes. The fish should look opaque and be the same color throughout. If it isn't, steam it again until it is cooked through.

**5** Mash the potatoes with 3 tablespoons of the milk and the spread. Purée the peas and fish together with the remaining milk, adding more if required, and mix together with the potatoes.

# Butterbean and sweet potato

A lovely introduction to beans, butterbeans taste fairly bland and combine nicely with the sweet potato and parsnips.

 5 mins  10–12 mins  5–6 portions

## ingredients

1¾oz (50g) **parsnips**, peeled and diced
3½oz (100g) **sweet potatoes**, peeled and diced
7oz (200g) can **butterbeans** in water,
drained and rinsed
a few sprigs of **parsley**, rinsed
1 tbsp **vegetable oil**
¼ cup cooled boiled **water** or **milk**

## method

**1** Place the parsnips and sweet potatoes in a steamer and cook for 5 minutes, or until almost tender.

**2** Add the butterbeans and parsley and steam for another 3–4 minutes to heat through.

**3** Purée with the oil and milk or water until smooth.

# Lentil, tomato, and coriander dhal

This simple dhal provides protein as well as iron and vitamin C for your baby. Serve it alone or thicken with rice cereal or mashed potatoes. As weaning progresses to include more lumpy food, you can mash rather than purée this dish.

 5 mins  20–25 mins

 4 portions

## ingredients

1 tbsp **vegetable oil**
scant 1oz (25g) **onions**, finely chopped
1¾oz (50g) split **red lentils**
7oz (200g) canned **tomatoes**, chopped
pinch of **ground coriander**
1 tsp chopped fresh **cilantro** (optional)

## method

**1** Heat the oil in a non-stick saucepan and cook the onion for 3–4 minutes until softened. Stir in the lentils, tomatoes, and ground coriander.

**2** Add ¾ cup of water and bring the mixture to a boil. Reduce the heat,
cover, and simmer for 15–20 minutes until the lentils are soft.

**3** Stir in the fresh cilantro and cook for another 1–2 minutes. Remove from the heat and cool slightly before puréeing.

**\*Tip:** If you are using fresh herbs, make sure that they are washed and patted dry on paper towels. Add green herbs in the last few minutes of cooking so that the heat destroys any food-poisoning bacteria.

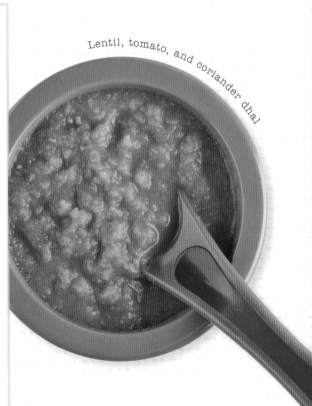

Lentil, tomato, and coriander dhal

Chicken and broccoli

# Chicken and broccoli

Your baby will already be familiar with broccoli; combining this with chicken provides a protein-rich meal. You can serve this dish on its own or thicken it with a little rice cereal to make a more complete meal.

🕐 5–6 mins          🔥 8–10 mins

🥧 6–8 portions       ❄️

## ingredients

1 tbsp **vegetable oil**
3½oz (100g) ground **chicken**

7oz (200g) **broccoli florets**
⅓ cup cooled and boiled **water** or **milk**

## method

**1** Heat the oil in a small pan and gently cook the chicken for 2 minutes before stirring in ¼ cup water.

**2** Cover and simmer for 5 minutes, or until the chicken is cooked through.

**3** Steam the broccoli florets until tender. Purée the chicken with any cooking liquid and add the broccoli. Blend with the remaining water or milk until smooth.

**✱ Tip:** *If you are adding rice cereal, mix in 1 heaping teaspoon of rice cereal for each tablespoon of the purée.*

# Beef, carrot, and potato

Beef is a good source of iron and zinc, so it is an important protein-rich food to introduce to your baby at around six months of age. Choose lean ground beef as this is lower in saturated fats, and cook it in healthy monounsaturated vegetable (canola) oil.

 5–10 mins    18–20 mins    8–10 portions

## ingredients

1 tbsp **vegetable oil**
3½oz (100g) **lean ground beef**
7oz (200g) **carrots**, peeled, quartered, and sliced
7oz (200g) **potatoes**, peeled and diced
**milk** to blend, if needed

## method

**1** Heat the oil in a saucepan and gently cook the beef for 2–3 minutes until lightly browned.

**2** Add the carrots to the beef along with ¾ cup water, and bring to a boil. Stir, cover, and reduce the heat. Allow to simmer for 15 minutes, or until the carrots are soft.

**3** Meanwhile, steam or boil the potatoes. Purée the carrots, beef, and cooking water until smooth.

**4** Press the cooked potatoes through a ricer or food mill, or mash finely using a little milk if needed. Mix the potatoes with the beef and carrots.

**✱ Tip:** *As the potato is cooked alone, you can freeze the beef and carrot mixture separately if you prefer. By pulsing the blender or processor, you can achieve a coarser purée, which is useful for stage 2 weaning.*

**✱ Variations:** *Use lamb instead of ground beef. Add ¼ teaspoon dried mixed herbs at stage 3.*

# Lamb and apricots

Lamb, like beef, provides easily absorbed iron and zinc. The addition of tomatoes here ensures there is vitamin C to help your baby absorb the iron. You can use this purée alongside mashed potatoes, with rice, or in the later stages of weaning with couscous.

 5 mins  15–20 mins  6–8 portions

## ingredients

3½oz (100g) ground **lamb**
1¾oz (50g) dried **apricots**, halved if large
7oz (200g) **tomato purée**
pinch of ground **cinnamon**

## method

**1** Place the lamb in a small non-stick saucepan and gently brown in its own fat over low heat for 2–3 minutes, stirring constantly to break up the lamb.

**2** Add the apricots, tomato purée, and ½ cup water. Sprinkle in the cinnamon, stir, and cover.

**3** Simmer gently for 10–15 minutes, stirring occasionally, until the lamb is cooked through and the apricots are tender. Cool the mixture slightly, then purée.

**4** Serve with rice cereal, potato, or sweet potato.

*★ Tip: You can use a 7oz (200g) can of chopped tomatoes in juice instead of tomato purée.*

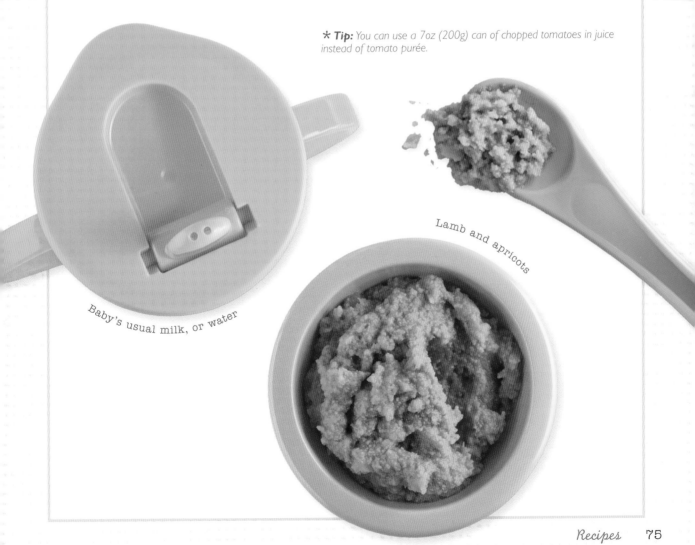

Baby's usual milk, or water

Lamb and apricots

# Introducing *Stage 2*

**In the second stage of weaning, around seven to nine months**, your baby's ability to grasp objects improves, and she may hold a spoon, pick up soft finger foods, and gets used to holding a spouted cup. She eats two to three meals a day, which play an increasingly important role nutritionally. As her muscles strengthen, she sits more upright in a high chair, giving her a good view of what's going on at mealtimes.

## Progressing through the second stage

The texture of your baby's meals changes during this stage from puréed food to mashed food (if you haven't done this already), food with soft lumps, and ground foods. She will also be eating a range of finger foods.

Her ability to chew improves during this stage, whether or not she has any teeth, so it's vital that she is introduced to lumps in food as well as dissolving or soft finger foods so she can practice chewing. Start by introducing soft lumps in familiar foods, such as well-cooked potatoes and vegetables. Tiny pasta shapes are also ideal lumpy foods that will encourage her to chew. She can progress onto larger lumps and slightly harder textures, including finger foods, over the weeks. Don't delay this phase for fear that she might choke: it's important for her to manage soft lumps by the time she is nine months old, otherwise she may become resistant to trying new textures if left too long.

Continuity and perseverance are important during this stage. Keep offering savory foods and vegetables in preference to desserts or fruit, so that your baby doesn't reject savory in favor of sweet.

## What your baby eats now

- Milk, whether breast or formula, is still vital to your baby. In this stage, as your baby starts to eat larger amounts of foods, the amount of milk she wants may go down a little, although she shouldn't have less than around 16oz (500ml), or two to four breastfeeds a day. If you decide to start weaning your baby from breastfeeding now, make sure you choose a suitable formula as an alternative (see p47).

- By this second stage of weaning, your baby should be eating meals that contain meat, fish, or poultry once a day. These provide essential protein, B vitamins, iron, zinc, and omega 3 fatty acids, which milk alone doesn't supply adequately for your growing baby. The menu plans will help you to introduce nutrient-rich foods such as lamb, chicken, beef, cod, salmon, and tofu.

- Vegetarian babies need a mixture of beans, tofu, nut and seed butters, and cheese to provide different vegetarian sources of protein. You could also talk to a pediatrician about giving an omega-3 supplement.

- Although milk is still vital, you may be giving other drinks, too; there's advice on pages 46-7 on which fluids are suitable for your baby.

## Timing meals and milk feeds

When your baby's daily meal quota goes up, you may need to alter the timing of her milk feeds so she has an appetite for food. Mornings are tricky as your baby wakes up hungry and may be used to a large milk feed. If this is her routine, you could give her a milk feed first thing, then delay her breakfast until you are up and ready for the day. If she has a large feed late morning, try splitting this so she has some before lunch and the rest after lunch (perhaps giving two smaller bottles or offering just one breast at a time). As you progress, you will probably find you develop a pattern of regular meals that fit around sleep and activities.

## STAGE 2 – at a glance

**TEXTURE**

During the second stage of weaning, the texture of your baby's food should progress from **mashed food** to **chopped textures** and **soft** or **dissolving** finger foods.

**INTRODUCE**

cow's milk in cooking · more pasta products · soft berries · soy and tofu products · eggs · nuts.* *Note, if you have a family history of allergies, consult your doctor before giving your baby nuts.

**AVOID**

Don't give processed meats, such as sausages and ham, honey, liver, and whole nuts (see p19).

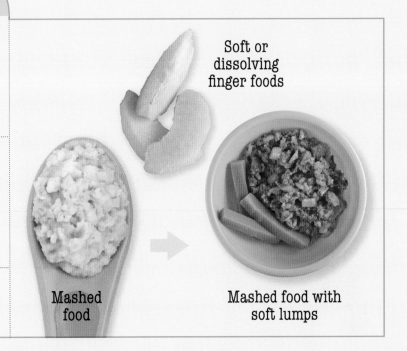

**Soft or dissolving finger foods**

**Mashed food**

**Mashed food with soft lumps**

## Portion sizes

The table below is a guide to the usual portion sizes for babies during stage 2, although individual babies will differ on the amount they need to eat. It assumes that foods from the main food groups are mixed together.

| FOODS | TYPICAL MEAL | TYPICAL AMOUNT FOR 7–9 MONTH OLD |
|---|---|---|
| Cereal mixed with milk | Breakfast | 5 teaspoons to 5 tablespoons per meal |
| Fruit purée with dairy | Dessert or breakfast | 5 teaspoons |
| Savory dish including vegetables, protein source (meat, poultry, fish, or beans) and pasta, potatoes, or rice | Lunch or dinner | 5–10 teaspoons per meal |
| Dairy—puddings or custards | Dessert – lunch or dinner | 5–10 teaspoons |
| Milk—formula or breastfeed | Throughout day | 16–20oz (500–600ml) formula (2–4 breastfeeds) |
| Finger foods | With meals | Half slice bread or 1 rice cake, or 2 pieces pasta, and 2–3 pieces softened fruit or vegetables |
| High-fat and high-sugar foods | Not suitable | Not suitable |

# Hands *on*

**Finger foods come into their own from stage 2 onward** as your baby's hand–eye coordination improves. Eating whole foods also helps her learn to chew efficiently, which in turn is an important part of speech development as she learns to coordinate the muscles needed for talking. Her control over her fingers and thumb improves now, so a chair with an attached tray is helpful as you can place finger foods right on the tray for her to attempt to grasp.

## Introducing finger foods

Soft fruits are perfect first finger foods, cut into pieces that are big enough for your baby to pick up and easy to eat. You may have already introduced these toward the end of stage 1, so can build on your baby's repertoire now. Make sure you remove any seeds or pits from fruits. You can also start to serve cooked vegetable finger foods alongside your baby's meals. Cut vegetables into batons, slices, or florets, and steam or oven bake them until soft. Over time, and as your baby's chewing skills develop, some of these can be introduced raw.

There are plenty of commercial baby snack foods that make great finger foods and can come in handy when you are out and about. However, try to resist the temptation to comfort or distract your baby at home with baby breadsticks and bite-and-dissolve snacks as these may spoil her appetite for meals.

## "I want to do it!"

Enjoying finger foods is an important part of learning to self-feed, giving your baby the chance to develop independent eating habits. If your baby was resistant to being spoon-fed, being able to feed herself finger foods allows her more control and can make mealtimes easier for you both. If you have followed the baby-led weaning route, you will have introduced finger foods from an earlier age, allowing your baby to select from a range of foods offered on her high-chair tray.

## Be careful

- Stay with your baby at all times when she is eating new textures and finger foods in case she chokes (see p39 on how to prepare foods to prevent choking).
- Be careful with dried fruit, as this can stick to teeth, increasing the risk of decay. Raisins are best left for mealtimes, unless you clean your baby's teeth afterward. You can soak dried fruit in a little water first to soften it.

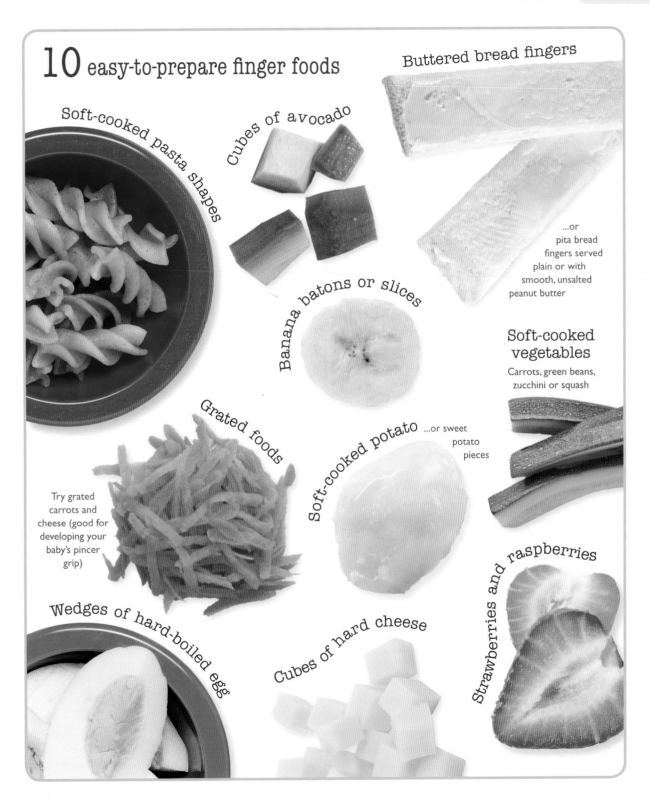

# 10 easy-to-prepare finger foods

Buttered bread fingers

Cubes of avocado

Soft-cooked pasta shapes

...or pita bread fingers served plain or with smooth, unsalted peanut butter

Banana batons or slices

## Soft-cooked vegetables

Carrots, green beans, zucchini or squash

Grated foods

Soft-cooked potato

...or sweet potato pieces

Try grated carrots and cheese (good for developing your baby's pincer grip)

Strawberries and raspberries

Wedges of hard-boiled egg

Cubes of hard cheese

# Eating *out*

**As you and your baby develop a routine**, you will be taking her out and about to meet friends and family, go shopping, or take trips to the park, which can mean being out during mealtimes. There are plenty of ideas for healthy, portable meals.

## Making the planner work away from home

The menu planner contains plenty of recipes that can be eaten cold. By swapping days around to suit your schedule, it's easy to make the planner work for you and your baby when you're away from home. Some portable foods include:

- Apricot and pear purée (p66)
- Avocado purée (p61)
- Banana purée (p59)
- Avocado and banana purée (p66)
- Homemade hummus (p111) with cooled steamed vegetables
- Cottage cheese dip (p107) with baby breadsticks or pita bread fingers
- Baby falafel (p110) with tzatziki

- Banana custard (p133)
- Creamy apricot dessert (p129)
- Stewed apples and cranberries (p129)

**As your baby grows and starts to eat more complete meals, you can try:**

- Baby pizzas (pp178–9)
- Fruity couscous (p189) and cottage cheese or cheese cubes
- Hard-boiled egg wedges (p69), cherry tomatoes, and bread and butter
- Baby blueberry pancakes (p169) spread with soft cheese
- Egg and sprouts sandwich (p175) with red bell pepper fingers
- Pasta – filled or plain
- Appley plums (p129)
- Rice pudding (p135) with mandarins

### *Staying safe*

When you're eating away from home, don't relax on safety and hygiene:

- Clean yours and your baby's hands before eating.
- When transporting homemade food, pack a bowl and several spoons so you can use one spoon for placing food in the bowl and the other spoon for feeding your baby. This ensures your baby's saliva doesn't contaminate food that hasn't been decanted.
- If you are using a jar of food, throw away any that remains uneaten if you can't refrigerate it—it isn't safe to use commercial food that has been opened and not eaten unless it is refrigerated right away.

- Don't give your baby a pouch of textured food to eat while she's sitting in her stroller. Your baby doesn't use her tongue to control food while sucking, so she is more likely to choke on a lump while sucking a pouch. Wait until you've stopped for lunch, then decant the pouch into a bowl.
- Never give your baby food to eat while you're driving unless there's an adult sitting next to her.

## Hot or cold?

If you wish to give your baby hot food away from home, you have a couple of options. You can cook and cool a meal, then reheat it at your destination, which works well if visiting friends. Or heat up food at home, then keep it warm in a wide-mouth flask.

Before adding food to the flask, rinse it out with boiling water and make sure the food has been heated until piping hot to keep bacteria from multiplying in warm conditions. If food needs to be kept cool, use a cool bag with a freezer block.

## Using store-bought foods

It's undoubtedly convenient to pack an unopened jar or pouch of baby food for days out, and shop-bought baby foods can add variety to your baby's diet. If an item is from the supermarket shelf rather than a fresh refrigerated food, it doesn't need special storage. It can be served at room temperature or, if you are in a restaurant or someone's home, you can ask for it to be heated.

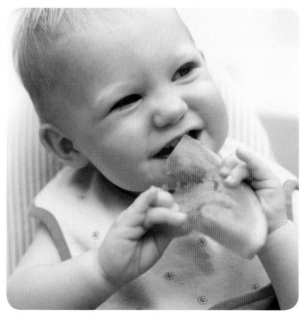

Easily transportable fruit is ideal for feeding away from home

## Eating in restaurants

Some restaurants are more baby-friendly than others, so it's worth finding out in advance what, if any, provision they make for little visitors. Check the following:

- Do they provide high chairs?

- Does the restaurant provide toys or crayons to keep older babies and children amused? If not, take some quiet toys along to keep her occupied; choose ones that will sit easily on the high-chair tray.

- Are there items on the menu that may be suitable for your baby, such as foods that you could mash with a fork or cut finely, or that she can pick up and eat herself? Avoid any food with added salt.

- If the restaurant doesn't have suitable foods on the menu, will they heat commercially bought baby food? (They are unlikely to heat homemade food because of the risk your food could pose.) Do they provide their own jars of baby food that they will heat up?

- Do they mind if you bring along some cold foods for your baby to eat at the table?

- Coffee shops rarely provide suitable foods for babies, so if you're planning to stop off at one on a trip out, take your own food or choose a simple sandwich.

# day-by-day meal planner
## Week 1

Offer your baby a drink with her meals. Either her usual milk or water in a lidded cup. If you wish to give juice, give unsweetened fruit juice diluted one part juice to 10 parts water.

## Monday

**Breakfast**
Apricot oatmeal p68

**Lunch**
Italian tomato and tuna mash p120

**Dinner**
Beef and onion casserole p116 with mashed potato
Banana custard p133

## Tuesday

**Breakfast**
Teething biscuit p70 with apple purée p59/milk

**Lunch**
Cod, pea, and potato p72

**Dinner**
Chicken and broccoli p74 with rice
Papaya fingers p131

## Wednesday

**Breakfast**
Millet and banana oatmeal p68

**Lunch**
Hard-boiled egg with buttered toast p69

**Dinner**
Cheesy mash with fish and peas p117
Creamy apricot dessert p129

## Thursday

**Breakfast**
Apricot and pear purée p66 with buttered toast p69

**Lunch**
Tofu and avocado dip p108

**Dinner**
Italian tomato and tuna mash p120
Yogurt with fruit purée p96

## Friday

**Breakfast**
Mango purée and yogurt p96

**Lunch**
Cheesy mash with fish and peas p117

**Dinner**
Yummy veggie sauce with pasta p122
Chocolate rice pudding p135

## Saturday

**Breakfast**
Apple and raspberries p97 with yogurt

**Lunch**
Homemade hummus p111 with steamed vegetables p118–19

**Dinner**
Lamb and apricots p75 with rice and cooked spinach
Stewed apple and cranberries p129

## Sunday

**Breakfast**
Banana oatmeal p68

**Lunch**
Beef and onion casserole p116 with mashed potato

**Dinner**
Creamy salmon and pasta p121
Fruit fool p133

**Other ideas this week** Raspberry porridge p99 • Carrot and lentil soup p103 • Sweet potato, barley, and leek soup p102 • Cauliflower cheese p125 with bread and butter • Fruity chicken p112 with mashed potato • Mango ice pops p132 • Halved grapes and pear slices p130

# day-by-day meal planner
## Week 2

## Monday

**Breakfast**
Greek yogurt and
sliced banana

**Lunch**
Homemade hummus p111
with steamed vegetables
pp118–19 and pita

**Dinner**
Lamb and apricots p75
with rice and broccoli
Fruit fool p133

## Tuesday

**Breakfast**
Banana oatmeal p68

**Lunch**
Hard-boiled egg with
buttered toast p69

**Dinner**
Fruity chicken p112 with
mashed sweet potato
Yogurt with fruit purée p96

## Wednesday

**Breakfast**
Teething biscuit p70 with
apple purée p59/milk

**Lunch**
Sweet potato, barley, and
leek soup p102

**Dinner**
Cod, pea, and potato p72
Ground rice
pudding p134

## Thursday

**Breakfast**
Yogurt and pear slices p130

**Lunch**
Chicken and broccoli p74
with rice

**Dinner**
Creamy salmon and
pasta p121
Fruit fool p133

## Friday

**Breakfast**
Millet oatmeal p68 with
apple purée p59

**Lunch**
Cottage cheese dip p107
with steamed vegetables
p118–19

**Dinner**
Coconut lentil dhal
p128 with rice
Berries with chocolate
dipping sauce p135

## Saturday

**Breakfast**
Spicy plum and banana p96

**Lunch**
Sweet potatoes with
sardines and peas p117

**Dinner**
Greek baked fish p120
with mashed potato
Soft pear slices p130

## Sunday

**Breakfast**
Date Oatmeal p98

**Lunch**
Avocado dip p105 with
bread

**Dinner**
Normandy pork p113
with mashed potato
Banana custard p133

---

*Other ideas this week* French toast p98 and fruit purée pp59–62 • Basic oatmeal p98 • Yummy veggie sauce with pasta p122 • Butternut squash risotto p122 • Beef ragu p115 with pasta shapes and broccoli florets • Garden vegetable risotto p127 • Appley plums p129

# day-by-day meal planner
# Week 3

## Monday

**Breakfast**
Hard-boiled egg with buttered toast p69

**Lunch**
Flaked fish p106 with avocado dip p105

**Dinner**
Tofu with spinach and rice p127
Mixed berry frozen yogurt p133

## Tuesday

**Breakfast**
Apricot and pear purée p66 with Greek yogurt

**Lunch**
Italian tomato and tuna mash p120

**Dinner**
Baby's first lamb tagine p115 with couscous p102
Fruit fool p133

## Wednesday

**Breakfast**
Date oatmeal p98 with pear slices p130

**Lunch**
Homemade hummus p111 with breadsticks/cucumber

**Dinner**
Fruity chicken p112 with mashed sweet potato
Canned peaches with semolina p134

## Thursday

**Breakfast**
Yogurt with strawberry slices p130

**Lunch**
Cod, pea, and potato p72

**Dinner**
Beef with prunes p116 with cooked spinach and rice
Stewed apple and cranberries p129

## Friday

**Breakfast**
Mango and vanilla p97

**Lunch**
Lentil and spinach dhal p128 with rice

**Dinner**
Creamy salmon and pasta p121
Rice pudding p135 with added dried fruit

## Saturday

**Breakfast**
Teething biscuits with fruit/milk p70

**Lunch**
Sweet potato, barley, and leek soup p102 with cheesy polenta "twigs" p108

**Dinner**
Cauliflower cheese p125
Papaya fingers p131

## Sunday

**Breakfast**
Millet and banana oatmeal p68

**Lunch**
Cheesy tomato risotto p124

**Dinner**
Creamy vegetable korma p126 with rice
Creamy apricot dessert p129

*Other ideas this week* Spicy banana toast p100 • Cheesy polenta "twigs" p108 with roasted Mediterranean vegetable dip p107 • Normandy pork p113 with mashed sweet potato and steamed green beans • Greek baked fish p120 with cooked spinach • Apple and pear fingers p130

# day-by-day meal planner
# Week 4

## Monday

**Breakfast**
Date oatmeal p98 and mango slices p131

**Lunch**
Flaked salmon p106 with avocado dip p105

**Dinner**
Vegetarian sauté p126 with rice
Berries with chocolate dipping sauce p135

## Tuesday

**Breakfast**
Toast and cream cheese p100
pear slices p130

**Lunch**
Butternut squash risotto p122

**Dinner**
Tofu with spinach and rice p127
Creamy apricot dessert p129

## Wednesday

**Breakfast**
Greek yogurt and mashed berries

**Lunch**
Hard-boiled egg with buttered toast p69 and bell pepper fingers

**Dinner**
Greek baked fish p120 with mashed potato
Stewed apple and cranberries p129

## Thursday

**Breakfast**
Spicy banana toast p100

**Lunch**
Tofu and avocado dip p108 with steamed carrot p118–19

**Dinner**
Baby's first lamb tagine p115 with couscous p102 and cooked spinach
Chocolate rice pudding p135

## Friday

**Breakfast**
Mango and vanilla p97

**Lunch**
Coconut lentil dhal p128 with rice

**Dinner**
Italian tomato and tuna mash p120
Banana with chocolate dipping sauce p135

## Saturday

**Breakfast**
French toast with strawberry slices p98

**Lunch**
Sweet potato, barley, and leek soup p112 with cheesy polenta "twigs" p108

**Dinner**
Chicken Provençale p112 with pasta shapes
Semolina p134 and apricot purée p60

## Sunday

**Breakfast**
Apple and raspberries p97

**Lunch**
Yummy veggie sauce with pasta p122 and grated cheese

**Dinner**
Beef with prunes p116 with broccoli and rice
Greek yogurt with fruit

*Other ideas this week* — Blueberry breakfast p97 • Toast and peanut butter p101 • Lentil and spinach dhal p128 • Steamed vegetable fingers pp118–19 with homemade hummus dip p111 • Garden vegetable risotto p127 • Herby lamb p114 with steamed greens and mashed potato • Fruit fool p133

# day-by-day meal planner
# Week

## Monday

### Breakfast
Teething biscuit p70 and banana slices

### Lunch
Carrot and lentil soup p103 with bread

### Dinner
Salmon and sweet potato cakes p121 with yogurt and green beans
Greek yogurt with fruit

## Tuesday

### Breakfast
French toast with fruit p98

### Lunch
Tuna dip p105 with breadsticks/raw or steamed vegetables pp118–19

### Dinner
Creamy vegetable korma p126 with rice
Mixed berry frozen yogurt p133

## Wednesday

### Breakfast
Millet oatmeal p68 with stewed fruit p129

### Lunch
Yummy veggie sauce with pasta and grated cheese p122

### Dinner
Normandy Pork p113 with mashed potato and broccoli
Yogurt with fruit purée p96

## Thursday

### Breakfast
Banana and kiwi p97

### Lunch
Scrambled egg p99 with toast and raw or steamed vegetables pp118–19

### Dinner
Vegetarian sauté p126 with couscous p102 and carrots
Fruit fool p133

## Friday

### Breakfast
Raspberry oatmeal p99

### Lunch
Italian tomato and tuna mash p120

### Dinner
Pork with pineapple p114 and steamed zucchini p118
Lemony ricotta pudding p134

## Saturday

### Breakfast
Yogurt with strawberry slices p130

### Lunch
Avocado dip p105 with steamed vegetables pp118–19 and breadsticks

### Dinner
Cheesy tomato risotto p124 and green beans
Appley plums p129

## Sunday

### Breakfast
Banana oatmeal p68

### Lunch
Mini lamb and mint balls p109 with avocado dip p105

### Dinner
Creamy salmon and pasta p121
Soft pear slices p130

*Other ideas this week* Mango and vanilla breakfast p97 • Cheese scones p104 with cottage cheese dip p107 • Sweet potato, barley, and leek soup p102 • Beef ragu p115 with pasta shapes and broccoli • Chicken and mushroom casserole p113 with mashed potato and green beans • Chocolate rice pudding p135

# day-by-day meal planner
## Week 6

## Monday

Breakfast
Blueberry and pear p97

Lunch
Carrot and lentil soup p103 with bread

Dinner
Pork with pineapple p114 with rice and broccoli
Ground rice pudding p134 with mashed berries

## Tuesday

Breakfast
Greek yogurt with banana slices

Lunch
Coconut lentil dhal p128 with rice

Dinner
Herby lamb with vegetables p114 and couscous p102
Stewed apple and raisins p129

## Wednesday

Breakfast
Toast and cream cheese p100 and halved grapes

Lunch
Scrambled egg p99 with toast/soft tomato pieces

Dinner
Cheesy tomato risotto p124 and corn
Creamy apricot dessert p129

## Thursday

Breakfast
Yogurt with whole raspberries

Lunch
Cauliflower cheese p125 and bread fingers

Dinner
Salmon and sweet potato cakes p121 with avocado dip p105 and green beans
Semolina p134 with fruit

## Friday

Breakfast
Bircher muesli p98

Lunch
Avocado dip p105 with dippers pp104–110

Dinner
Beef with prunes p116 with potatoes and broccoli
Yogurt with fruit purée p96

## Saturday

Breakfast
Scrambled egg p99 with toast

Lunch
Sweet potato, barley, and leek soup p102

Dinner
Chicken Provençale p112 with mashed potato
Fruit fool p133

## Sunday

Breakfast
Spicy banana toast p100

Lunch
Italian tomato and tuna mash p120 with cooked spinach

Dinner
Macaroni cheese p125 and steamed vegetables pp118–19
Mango ice pop p132

*Other ideas this week*  Date oatmeal p98 • Toast and peanut butter p101 • Broccoli cheese p125 with bread fingers • Baby falafel p110 with homemade hummus p111 • Baby's first vegetable curry p123 with rice • Avocado slices with toast fingers • Fruity chicken p112 with mashed potato • Appley plums p129

# day-by-day meal planner

## Week 7

### Monday

**Breakfast**
Bircher muesli p98

**Lunch**
Cauliflower cheese p125
and bread fingers

**Dinner**
Herby lamb with vegetables
p114 with
couscous p102
Berries with chocolate
dipping sauce p135

### Tuesday

**Breakfast**
Mango and vanilla p97

**Lunch**
Homemade hummus p111
with pita bread and pepper
fingers

**Dinner**
Beef ragu p115 with pasta
and zucchini p118
Mango ice pop p132

### Wednesday

**Breakfast**
Raspberry oatmeal p99

**Lunch**
Italian tomato and tuna
mash p120 with cooked
spinach

**Dinner**
Butternut squash risotto
p122 with green beans
Banana custard p133

### Thursday

**Breakfast**
Toast and cream cheese
p100 and halved grapes

**Lunch**
Carrot and lentil soup p103
with cheese scones p104

**Dinner**
Baby's first vegetable curry
p123 with chapati fingers
Greek yogurt with fruit

### Friday

**Breakfast**
Teething biscuit p70 with
milk and mashed
blueberries

**Lunch**
Cottage cheese dip p107
with rice cakes

**Dinner**
Greek baked fish p120 with
mashed potato and zucchini
Soft pear slices p130

### Saturday

**Breakfast**
Stewed fruit p129 and
yogurt with spoon of muesli

**Lunch**
Baby falafel p110 with
roasted Mediterranean
vegetable dip p107

**Dinner**
Normandy Pork p113 with
broccoli and baby pasta
Fruit fool p133

### Sunday

**Breakfast**
Bircher muesli p98

**Lunch**
Broccoli cheese p125 with
bread fingers

**Dinner**
Lentil and spinach
dhal p128 with rice
Yogurt with fruit purée p96

---

**Other ideas this week** Spicy plum and banana breakfast p96 • Flaked fish p106 with avocado dip p105 • Sweet potatoes with sardines and peas p117 • Chicken Provençale p112 with mashed potatoes and broccoli florets • Macaroni cheese p125 • Stewed apple and cranberries p129

# day-by-day meal planner

## Week 8

---

## Monday

**Breakfast**
Spicy banana toast p100

**Lunch**
Penne pasta with roasted Mediterranean vegetable dip p107

**Dinner**
Herby lamb with vegetables p114 and mashed potatoes
Yogurt with fruit purée p96

## Tuesday

**Breakfast**
Raspberry oatmeal p99

**Lunch**
Tuna dip p105 on toast with halved cherry tomatoes

**Dinner**
Beef and onion casserole p116 with mashed root vegetables
Chocolate rice pudding p135 and orange pieces

## Wednesday

**Breakfast**
Bircher muesli p98

**Lunch**
Creamy vegetable korma p126 with rice

**Dinner**
Greek baked fish p120 with mashed potatoes and green beans
Mango ice pop p132

## Thursday

**Breakfast**
Apricot oatmeal p68

**Lunch**
Italian tomato and tuna mash p120

**Dinner**
Pork with pineapple p114 with rice and cooked spinach
Mixed berry frozen yogurt p133

---

## Friday

**Breakfast**
Blueberry and pear p97

**Lunch**
Mini lamb and mint balls p109 with roasted Mediterranean vegetable dip p107

**Dinner**
Garden vegetable risotto p127
Papaya fingers p131

## Saturday

**Breakfast**
Toast and cream cheese p100 and canned peach slices

**Lunch**
Tofu and avocado dip p108 with breadsticks/steamed or raw vegetables pp118–19

**Dinner**
Chicken Provençale p112 with mashed vegetables
Yogurt with stewed fruit p129

## Sunday

**Breakfast**
Cinnamon spice pancakes p99

**Lunch**
Flaked salmon p106 with avocado dip p105 and bread and butter

**Dinner**
Beef with prunes p116 with cooked spinach and rice
Semolina p134 and apricot purée p60

---

**Other ideas this week**
Strawberry Greek yogurt p96 • Toast fingers p69 with cottage cheese dip p107 • Carrot and lentil soup p103 with cheese scones p104 • Cauliflower cheese p125 with toast fingers p69 • Tofu with spinach and rice p127 • Peach and nectarine slices p131

# day-by-day meal planner
# Week 9

By the end of stage 2, your baby has experienced many new tastes and is learning to chew more challenging textures.

## Monday

**Breakfast**
Yogurt with mango slices p131

**Lunch**
Tuna dip p105 on toast with halved cherry tomatoes

**Dinner**
Creamy vegetable korma p126 with rice
Fruit fool p133

## Tuesday

**Breakfast**
Basic oatmeal with banana slices p98

**Lunch**
Baby falafel p110 with yogurt and raw or steamed carrot sticks pp118–19

**Dinner**
Beef ragu p115 with pasta shapes and broccoli
Mango slices p131

## Wednesday

**Breakfast**
Cinnamon spice pancakes p99

**Lunch**
Carrot and lentil soup p103 with cheese scones p104

**Dinner**
Fruity chicken p112 with mashed potato and cooked spinach
Yogurt with mashed fruit

## Thursday

**Breakfast**
Bircher muesli p98

**Lunch**
Little sausage and apple balls p106 with apple purée dip p59 and bread

**Dinner**
Cauliflower or broccoli and cheese p125
Sliced pear or apple p130

## Friday

**Breakfast**
Teething biscuit with milk p70 and raisins

**Lunch**
Garden vegetable risotto p127

**Dinner**
Salmon and sweet potato cakes p121 with avocado dip p105
Strawberry or kiwi slices p130

## Saturday

**Breakfast**
Strawberry slices p130 and Greek yogurt

**Lunch**
Roasted Mediterranean vegetable dip p107 with pasta

**Dinner**
Chicken Provençale p112 with rice
Banana with chocolate dipping sauce p135

## Sunday

**Breakfast**
Spicy plum and banana p96

**Lunch**
Salmon and sweet potato cakes p121 with broccoli

**Dinner**
Herby lamb with vegetables p114 and couscous p102
Stewed apple and raisins p129

*Other ideas this week* Apple and raspberry breakfast p97 • Hard-boiled egg and buttered toast p69 • Sweet potatoes with sardines and peas p117 • Ratatouille p124 • Chicken and mushroom casserole p113 • Semolina pudding p134 with stewed fruit p129

# Tailor-made days

**As you become more practiced and confident** about preparing nutritious meals for your baby, you may find you have days when you want to tailor the meal plans to suit your own lifestyle. We all have times when the meals we cook are shaped by how demanding our day is, or which ingredients we have on hand. On some days, especially those when your baby wakes up fussy or clingy, time to cook is in short supply; whereas on others, time spent in the kitchen is soothing and satisfying. As you move into stage 3 of weaning, the top 10s that follow can help you tailor the odd day in the meal plans to suit your requirements.

## Meals for leisurely days

Slow-cooking dishes or ones that involve a bit more preparation are perfect for at-home days when you have more time on your hands. The longer cooking times for some of these meals also free up time for you to spend with your baby and get household chores done while dinner takes care of itself.

Slowly stewed meat is infused with flavors and deliciously tender, making it easy for your baby to chew.

1 Sweet potato, barley, and leek soup p102

2 Butternut/pumpkin and tomato soup p180

3 Normandy pork p113

4 Baby's first lamb tagine p115

5 Beef and onion casserole p116

6 Beef with prunes p116

7 Cheesy tomato risotto p124

8 Ratatouille p124

9 Garden vegetable risotto p127

10 Vegetarian shepherd's pie p189

Certain foods benefit nutritionally from longer cooking times. Tomatoes release more of the protective antioxidant lycopene during the cooking process.

And dessert:

· Rice pudding p135

· Baked stuffed apple p190

· Pear and raisin oat crumble p193

Garden vegetable risotto

# Meals for busy days

The recipes here are spot on for days when you've been out and about and have little time left for cooking. Quick to rustle up, each dish has nutritional value, too. If you know certain days will be a little hectic, buy core fresh ingredients such as fish or chicken ahead for the fridge or freezer to reach for when needed.

**1** Pesto, tomato, and mozzarella pizza p178

**2** Pea and mint soup p181

**3** Fruity chicken p112

**4** Chicken and pasta with creamy sauce p183

**5** Pork with pineapple p114

**6** Cheesy mash with fish and peas p117

**7** Greek baked fish p120

**8** Cauliflower/broccoli and cheese p125

**9** Vegetarian sauté p126

**10** Creamy avocado pasta p188

And dessert:

· Creamy apricot dessert p129

· Fresh fruit pp130–31

· Exotic fruit salad p191

· Passion fruit and mango dessert p191

Shorter cooking times preserve more of the essential vitamins B and C, making quick-cook dishes convenient and healthy.

Commercially frozen vegetables often provide as much vitamin C as their fresh equivalents, and are a godsend on days when you're pressed for time.

Pesto, tomato, and mozzarella pizza

## Pantry recipes

For days when fresh supplies are running low and you can't get to the store, a well-stocked cupboard and some core fridge items offer some great meal solutions. The recipes below provide some delicious meals and lighter bites that can be easily prepared from storecupboard basics.

**1** Cheese scones p104

**2** Polenta twigs p108 with tuna dip p105

**3** Scrambled eggs p99

**4** Sardines/beans on toast p173

**5** Italian tomato and tuna mash p120

**6** Macaroni and cheese p125

**7** Tofu with spinach and rice p127

**8** Coconut lentil dhal p128

**9** Cowboy beans with cornmeal topping p188

**10** Fruity couscous with peanut sauce p189

And dessert:

· Mixed berry frozen yogurt p133

· Semolina pudding p134

· Bread and butter pudding p194

· Baked egg custard p195

*Italian tomato and tuna mash*

Pasta, rice, and couscous are core staples for your pantry, providing a starchy base for many dishes.

Canned beans provide protein and are super convenient: most require heating just briefly before adding to dishes, avoiding the more lengthy soaking process needed for dried beans.

*Mixed berry frozen yogurt*

# Economy dishes

As food prices rise, we are all a bit more conscious of what goes on the weekly grocery list. The good news is that being economical doesn't have to equal less healthy eating. For weeks when you want to cut down a little on more costly meat and fish dishes, recipes using beans, hearty soups, and simple pasta dishes all provide filling, nutritious, and cost-effective meals.

1 Carrot and lentil soup p103

2 Baked potato with Mexican beans p177

3 Mushroom and onion pizza p178

4 Leek and potato soup p180

5 Italian tomato and tuna mash p120

6 Butternut squash risotto p122

7 Baby's first vegetable curry p123

8 Macaroni and cheese p125

9 Lentil and spinach dhal p128

10 Vegetarian shepherd's pie p189

And dessert:

• Appley plums p129

• Banana custard p133

• Semolina p134

• Baked spiced peach p190

Baked potatoes are nutritious, versatile—being the perfect base for a variety of delicious toppings,—and a great source of energy.

Mexican beans

Vegetables and fruits are cheaper in season, when they also tend to be more nutritious.

*Tailor-made days*   95

# Ways with *purées*

**Purées are a great introduction to solids,** getting your baby used to new tastes and textures. As weaning progresses and your baby's repertoire of foods expands, purées continue to be a useful way to include fruits and vegetables in her diet, whether as an addition to breakfasts and desserts or a topping for toast.

### Apricot yogurt breakfast

Mix 1 tablespoon of apricot purée (p60) with 1 tablespoon of full-fat yogurt.

### Spicy peach breakfast

Mix a pinch of cinnamon with 1 tablespoon of peach purée (p61), and stir into 1 tablespoon of full-fat Greek yogurt.

*Natural yogurt*

*Spicy peach breakfast*

### Spicy plum and banana breakfast

Stew 2 small ripe plums, which you have washed and quartered, in 1 tbsp water until they are soft. Blend until smooth. Mash half a small banana and stir in the plum purée along with a pinch of apple pie spice.

### Strawberries and yogurt

Wash and hull 2 medium ripe strawberries. Mash well with a fork until smooth, and stir into 1 heaping tablespoon of full-fat Greek yogurt.

## With crêpes!

### Blueberry breakfast

Mix 1 tablespoon of blueberry purée (p60) with 1 tablespoon of full-fat Greek yogurt.

### Apple and raspberry breakfast

Take 3–4 fresh or defrosted raspberries and mash into 1 tablespoon of apple purée (p59).

### Blueberry and pear breakfast

Mix 1 tablespoon of blueberry purée (p60) with 1 tablespoon of pear purée (p59).

## With toast

## With Greek yogurt

### Banana and kiwi breakfast

Peel and halve a ripe kiwi fruit, removing the white core, and mash well with a fork. Mash half a small banana and mix with the kiwi.

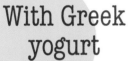

### Mango and vanilla breakfast

Mix 1 tablespoon of mango purée (p59) with 2 drops of vanilla extract and combine with 1 tablespoon of full-fat Greek yogurt.

## With cereals

Oatmeal

# Bircher muesli

This Swiss-derived muesli uses grated apples and juice and is soaked overnight in the fridge, which softens all the ingredients. It makes a delicious and healthy start to the day, so make a batch for both you and your baby.

 5 mins  Soaking time: overnight  1 baby and 1 adult portion ❄

## ingredients

1 heaping tbsp **rolled oats**
1 medium **apple**,
  peeled, cored, and grated
3 tbsp **orange juice**
3 heaping tbsp
  **full-fat natural yogurt**
pinch of **apple pie spice**
**raisins** (optional)

## method

**1** Blend the oats and process until fine. Place in a bowl.

**2** Add all the other ingredients, except the raisins and mix well. Cover with plastic wrap and refrigerate overnight.

**3** Stir a few raisins into your portion, if you like, but do not add any to your baby's portion until they are used to chewing more solid food.

\*Serve *with mashed blueberries or a few slices of banana.*
\*Store *in the refrigerator in an airtight container for up to 48 hours.*
\*Variations: *Add 1 teaspoon of ground almonds or unsweetened coconut in step 1. As your baby becomes more used to chewing, omit step 1.*

# French toast with fruit

French toast makes a nutritious start to the day. This recipe uses a slice of brioche, which is soft and enriched with milk and eggs. Serve with any fruit: slices of kiwi or soft pear or blueberries. Your baby only needs half an egg, so this makes enough for two.

 5 mins  1 baby and 1 adult portion

 4–6 mins

## ingredients

1 **egg**
1–2 tsp **butter**
  **or olive oil**

2–3 small slices of
  **brioche loaf**
**fruit** of choice, to serve

## method

**1** Beat the egg in a shallow dish or plate.

**2** Heat the butter or oil in a non-stick frying pan. Dip a slice of brioche into the beaten egg and quickly turn it over with a fork or tongs to coat the other side.

**3** Cook for a minute on each side until lightly browned.

**4** Cool a little and cut into bite-sized pieces for your baby. Serve with fruit.

\* *Not suitable for storing.*

# Basic oatmeal

Rolled oats, sometimes called old fashioned oats, cook more quickly than steel cut oats and provide soluble fiber, which has many health benefits.

 1 min  2–3 mins ◔ 1 portion

## ingredients

2 tbsp **rolled oats**          ²/₃ cup **whole milk**

## method

**1** Place the oats and milk in a small pan and heat, stirring continuously.

**2** When the mixture thickens, remove from the heat. Cool to body temperature and serve.

\* Microwave version: *Mix the oats and milk in a bowl and cook on high for 30 seconds (800W oven). Stir and cook for another 10 seconds. (The timing will vary according to the power of your oven.) Once thickened, remove and cool.*

\* Variations: *You can add ½oz (15g) of dried, semi-dried or fresh dates. Dates provide natural sweetness as well as dietary fiber. If using dried chopped dates, you may need to soak them in hot water for 10 minutes before use, to soften them. If using fresh dates, peel off the skin, remove the pit, and then chop. Similarly, if using semi-dried dates, remove the pit and chop.*

# Raspberry oatmeal

A lovely pink oatmeal, this is quick to make and will go down quickly as well.

 1 min    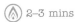 2–3 mins    1 portion

## ingredients

2 tbsp **rolled oats**
⅔ cup **whole milk**

4–5 **raspberries**, fresh, or frozen and defrosted

## method

**1** Place the oats and milk in a small pan and heat, stirring continuously.

**2** When the mixture thickens, add the raspberries and stir in

well so that the fruit breaks up.

**3** Remove from the heat and cool to body temperature before serving.

✳ Microwave version: *Mix oats and milk in a microwaveable bowl and cook on high for 30 seconds (800W oven). Stir and cook for 10 seconds. (Timing varies according to the microwave's power.) Once thickened, remove, add the raspberries, and cool.*

# Scrambled eggs

An easy, nutritious breakfast, scrambled eggs provide protein, iron, and vitamins A and D. Depending on your baby's appetite, you may need to help her eat this. Or use two larger eggs and have some, too.

 2 mins     2 mins     1–2 portions

## ingredients

1 **egg**
2 tbsp **whole milk**

1 tsp **olive oil spread**

## method

**1** In a small bowl, beat together the egg and milk.

**2** Heat the spread in a small saucepan and when melted stir in the egg mixture.

**3** Cook over low heat until the egg just thickens.

**4** Spoon into a bowl and let cool to body temperature.

**5** Serve with toast fingers.

# Cinnamon spice pancakes

These silver dollar pancakes provide your baby with a nice introduction to warm spices like cinnamon and nutmeg. A handy snack, these are also a good finger food addition to fruit at breakfast.

 5 mins     10–15 mins     16 drop scones    ✳

## ingredients

½ cup **whole milk**
1 **egg**
½ cup **self-rising flour**
½ cup **whole wheat flour**

1 tbsp **maple syrup** or 2 tsp sugar
¼ tsp **apple pie spice**
1 tbsp **vegetable oil**, for greasing

## method

**1** Place a griddle or non-stick frying pan over medium–high heat.

**2** Meanwhile, blend all the ingredients, except the oil until you have a thick batter.

**3** Brush the pan or griddle lightly with oil

and spoon a few teaspoonfuls of batter into the pan to make individual pancakes. Cook 1 minute on one side, then carefully turn over to cook the other side. When fully cooked, remove from the pan and cool slightly before serving or storing.

*Cinnamon spice pancakes*

✳ **Serve** *with cream cheese, butter, or spread. These can also be served with a fruit purée (see pp59–62).*

✳ **Store** *in the refrigerator for up to 24 hours, or freeze when cool.*

✳ **Variations:** *Once your baby can chew more efficiently, try adding a handful of raisins to the mixture after blending.*

# Ways with *toast*

**Toast makes an easy breakfast** as your baby can self feed, and by the end of this stage, she will be quite adept at coping with finger foods. It's important not to rely on buttered toast alone, as your baby needs protein (dairy or meat) and fruit, too.

## Spicy banana toast

This fruity addition to your baby's toast fingers provides essential vitamins and slow-release energy to keep her going through the morning.

### ingredients

½ slice of **white bread**
**butter** or
**monounsaturated**
**spread**

pinch of **cinnamon**
few slices of **banana**

### method

**1** Toast the bread lightly and spread the butter over it.

**2** Sprinkle with the cinnamon and cut into bite-sized pieces.

**3** Place the banana slices on top and serve.

## Toast and cream cheese

Cream cheese provides less protein than cottage cheese, but is fine to use occasionally. Your baby doesn't need the low-fat varieties of cream cheese, so if you are buying for the family, make sure hers is full-fat.

### method

**1** Any type of bread without hard seeds or grains is fine—try white, whole wheat, or brioche bread. Toast the bread lightly and spread approximately 1 tablespoon of cream cheese per slice.

A portion for a baby of 7–9 months is ½–1 small slice.

**2** Serve with sliced strawberries or kiwi fruit. For an older baby, try raw red bell pepper pieces or halved, seeded cherry tomatoes.

Cream cheese

# Toast and peanut butter

Use low-salt and low-sugar peanut butter, and a smooth variety as crunchy ones can cause choking. If allergies run in the family, consult your doctor before giving your baby peanut butter.

## method

**1** You can use white or whole wheat bread, or try with pita bread. Toast the bread lightly and spread approximately 1 tablespoon of peanut butter a slice. A portion for a 7–9 month-old baby is ½–1 small slice.

**2** Serve with sliced bananas or halved blueberries. For an older baby, serve with raw cucumber pieces.

Couscous

# Couscous

This very easy starchy accompaniment is enjoyed by babies as it is soft, and by parents as it doesn't require much effort to make! It is available whole wheat or plain, and with large or small grains; this recipe uses the most commonly found small-grained plain type.

 1 min       1 baby portion

5 mins      ❄️

## ingredients

1 tbsp **couscous**

## method

**1** Place the couscous in a small ramekin or bowl and pour in 2 tablespoons of boiling water. Stir and let stand for 5 minutes.

**2** Fluff with a fork and serve.

✳ **Variations:** *Add 1 teaspoon of olive oil with the water. For citrus couscous use 1 tablespoon of boiling water and 1 tablespoon of freshly squeezed orange juice.*

# Sweet potato, barley, and leek soup

Sweet potatoes make delicious soups, as well as provide a huge boost of vitamin A. Adults, babies, and children will enjoy this mild sweet soup, and it is worth making a double batch so you can freeze it for a cold day, when it makes a welcoming warm lunch. Fresh stock improves the flavor, but don't add salted stock to your baby's food.

 15 mins    40–45 mins    3–4 baby and 3 generous adult portions    ❄️

## ingredients

1 tbsp **olive oil**
6oz (175g) **leeks**, sliced finely
5½oz (150g) **carrots**, peeled and diced
7oz (200g) **sweet potatoes**, peeled and diced
2½ cups salt-free **vegetable** or **chicken stock**
1¾oz (50g) **pearl barley**
3 **bay leaves**
a few **parsley stems** (optional)
**salt** and **pepper**, to taste

## method

**1** Heat the oil in a non-stick saucepan and gently cook the leeks for 5 minutes, softening, but not browning it. Add the carrots and sweet potatoes, stir, and cover. Sweat the vegetables for another 5 minutes.

**2** Add the stock, barley, bay leaves, and parsley. Bring to a boil, stir, cover, and simmer for 30–35 minutes, stirring occasionally.

**3** Remove the bay leaves and the parsley. Add the parsley to the mixture to be blended.

**4** Let cool slightly, then blend half the soup and mix with the remaining soup.

**5** Remove your baby's portion, blend further, if needed, and serve at body temperature. Season your portion, adding salt and pepper as needed, and serve.

✳ **Serve** *with Cheese scones (see p104), bread, or rolls.*

✳ **Refrigerate** *in an airtight container for up to 24 hours or freeze when cool.*

✳ **Variations:** *A large onion can be used instead of the leek.*

# Carrot and lentil soup

This simple soup uses wholesome inexpensive ingredients that both you and your baby can enjoy together. Offer a couple of tablespoons of soup in her bowl and allow her to enjoy dipping a few fingers of toast or bread into it. You can then spoon-feed more to her as required.

 5 mins       25–30 mins       2 baby and 2 generous adult portions

## ingredients

1 tbsp **vegetable oil**, for cooking
3½oz (100g) or 1 small **leek**, finely sliced
9oz (250g) **carrots**, peeled and diced
5½oz (150g) **celeriac** or **rutabaga**, peeled and diced
1¾oz (50g) **split red lentils**
2½ cups salt free **vegetable or chicken stock**
1 **bay leaf**
**salt** and **black pepper**, to taste
pinch of **grated nutmeg**, to serve

✱ **Serve** *with pieces of whole wheat or white toast.*

✱ **Refrigerate** *in an airtight container for up to 24 hours or freeze when cool.*

✱ **Variations:** *Celery can be used, but as it can be fibrous, it is recommended that the soup be puréed well to avoid stringy parts remaining.*

## method

**1** Heat the oil in a large non-stick saucepan and gently cook the leeks for 3–4 minutes until soft. Add the carrots and celeriac, stir, cover, and sweat for 5 minutes without browning the vegetables.

**2** Stir in the lentils, stock, and bay leaf and bring to a boil, stirring occasionally.

**3** Cover, reduce the heat, and simmer for 15–20 minutes, or until the vegetables are tender and the lentils have become soft. Take off the heat and remove the bay leaf.

**4** Remove a portion for your baby and allow to cool a little before processing to a suitable texture. Pour into your baby's bowl and let cool to body temperature before serving.

**5** Meanwhile, for your portion, adjust the seasoning in the remainder of the soup, adding a little salt and black pepper as desired. If you like a chunky soup, process half the soup until smooth and mix with the rest of it in the pan. If you prefer a smoother soup, blend the whole portion.

**6** Pour into a bowl and grate over a pinch of nutmeg.

Carrot and lentil soup

# Dips and *dippers*

**For babies who like to self-feed,** homemade dips can be an easy way of providing protein and vegetables, and there are lots of interesting things to serve them with. As well as breadsticks, rice cakes, and crackers, try the dippers suggested here. Dips are best made and served fresh as most don't freeze well.

## Cheese scones

Little cheese scones can be made in a jiffy and taste great with soup, as well as being handy for breakfast or a quick snack. Use sharp Cheddar so you can taste the cheese.

 10 mins      12–15 mins      10–12 small scones

### ingredients

- 1 cup **whole wheat flour**
- 1 cup **all-purpose flour**, plus extra for dusting
- 3 tsp **baking powder**
- 2 tbsp **full-fat butter** or **spread**
- 1¾oz (50g) **Cheddar cheese**, grated
- ⅔ cup **whole milk**, plus extra for brushing

### method

**1** Preheat the oven to 400°F (200°C).

**2** Sift the flours and baking powder into a bowl, adding back any bran that remains. Rub the butter into the flour and stir in the grated cheese.

**3** Using a small palette or round-ended knife, stir the milk into the dry ingredients until you have a soft, but not sticky, mixture. Press the mixture into a ball. Sprinkle a little flour on a clean cutting board or work surface and roll out, or gently press the dough to around ½in (1.5cm) thick.

**4** Place a baking sheet in the hot oven for a couple of minutes.

**5** Using 1½–2in (4–5cm) cutters, stamp out scones until the dough is used up, gently re-rolling unused dough.

**6** Carefully place the scones on the hot baking sheet and brush the tops with a little milk. Bake for 12–15 minutes, or until the scones are risen and golden. Cool and serve fresh.

\* **Serve** *with creamy cheese or monounsaturated spread. These are also delicious with soup, or dips and vegetable sticks.*

\* *These are best eaten on the day they are made. Refrigerate in an airtight container for up to 24 hours or freeze when cool.*

\* **Variations:** *Replace the whole wheat flour with white flour.*

# Avocado dip

Avocados are a good source of protective vitamin E as well as healthy monounsaturated fats. Simply mash with a little lemon juice to prevent browning, and add in other ingredients as you wish to introduce new flavors and textures.

 5 mins    1 baby and 1 adult portion

## ingredients

1 ripe **avocado**, halved and pit removed
juice of ½ **lemon**

### Optional additions to make guacamole:

1 ripe **tomato**, peeled, seeded, and finely chopped
1 **scallion**, trimmed and finely chopped (once your baby can chew properly)
few drops **Tabasco sauce**

## method

**1** Scoop out the avocado flesh from the shell and mash until smooth with the lemon juice.

**2** Serve at once, or add other ingredients to make guacamole.

✳ **Serve** *with Flaked fish (see p106), steamed vegetable pieces (raw for older babies), baby breadsticks, or pieces of pita bread. Alternatively, use as a filling for sandwiches.*

✳ *Not suitable for storing.*

Avocado dip

# Tuna dip

Tuna is a pantry essential, and is often well accepted by babies. However, the canning process destroys most of the important omega-3 fatty acids, so don't rely exclusively on tuna as an oily fish; try salmon and sardines in your baby's diet, too. This dip is simple to make and has lots of variations.

 5 mins    2 baby and 2 adult portions

## ingredients

2½oz (70g), or ½ can, **tuna** in oil, drained
1¾oz (50g) **full-fat cream cheese**
1 tsp **tomato paste**
finely grated zest of half small **lemon**
½ tsp finely chopped **dill**

## method

**1** Process all the ingredients until smooth.

**2** Spoon into a small container(s). Cover and chill until required.

✳ **Serve** *with baby breadsticks, pieces of cucumber or pepper, or cooked carrot and green beans.*

# Little sausage and apple balls

Using premium quality sausages and fresh apple, these little balls are ideal for small hands to hold for self-feeding. They are quick to make and freeze well. Pork is a great source of vitamin B1 (thiamine).

 5 mins    15–20 mins    6–7 small balls   ❄

## ingredients

2oz (65g) or 1 premium quality **sausage**, peeled

½ medium **apple**, peeled and coarsely grated

3 tbsp fresh **bread crumbs**

## method

**1** Preheat the oven to 375°F (190°C).

**2** Process all the ingredients or mix together with a fork until well combined. Shape into balls around the size of an unshelled walnut.

**3** Place on a greased baking sheet and bake in the oven for 15–20 minutes, or until the center is piping hot and cooked through. Let cool before serving.

＊**Serve** *with a dip, such as Roasted Mediterranean vegetable dip (see opposite) or Avocado dip (see p105).*

＊**Refrigerate** *in an airtight container for up to 48 hours, or freeze when cool.*

＊**Variations:** *Instead of baking in the oven, cook in 1 tablespoon of vegetable oil, browning on all sides. Drain on paper towels.*

# Flaked fish

A white fish such as cod or a thick piece of salmon has large flakes that a baby can hold and eat. These are great for dipping in tomato salsa or other dips. Choose a thick piece of fish fillet, weighing around 3½oz (100g), and run your finger over the flesh to check for any bones, removing any you find. Bake, steam, or microwave until the fish is opaque. When you press it, it should gently break into flakes. Cool a little, remove the skin, and then give your baby a few flakes to enjoy.

## method

**Bake**
Bake at 350°F (180°C) for 15 minutes.

or

**Steam**
Wrap in foil or parchment paper and steam for 8–10 minutes.

or

**Microwave**
Microwave on high for 3–5 minutes depending on the power of the microwave.

Flaked fish

# Roasted Mediterranean vegetable dip

Rich in vitamins C and A, this sweet dip is great for dipping vegetables or baby breadsticks. Alternatively, it can be used as a sandwich filling.

 5 mins     25–30 mins    1 baby and 1 adult portion

## ingredients

1 **red bell pepper**, cut into large chunks
6 ripe **cherry tomatoes**, halved
1 small **red onion**, peeled and chopped
1–2 tbsp **olive oil**
5 large **basil leaves**, torn into 2 or 3 pieces
3½oz (100g) **mascarpone cheese**
2 tsp lemon juice

## method

**1** Preheat the oven to 400°F (200°C).

**2** Place the bell pepper, tomatoes, and onion in a roasting pan, drizzle with the oil, and roast in the oven for 25–30 minutes, or until the vegetables are soft.

✱ Serve *with Cheesy polenta "twigs" (see p108) or Mini lamb and mint balls (see p109).*

**3** Let cool for a few minutes, then blend until smooth. Add the basil, mascarpone, and lemon juice, and pulse lightly to mix. Chill until required.

*Roasted Mediterranean vegetable dip*

# Cottage cheese dip

Richer in protein and calcium than cream cheese or yogurt, cottage cheese blends to a smooth consistency, making simple dips and easy sandwich spreads for your baby.

 5 mins     1 min     2 baby and 1 adult portion

## ingredients

3½oz (100g), or 2 ripe medium **tomatoes**
**full-fat plain cottage cheese**

scant 1oz (25g) **Cheddar cheese**, grated
2 tsp **chives**, washed and snipped

## method

**1** Peel the tomatoes by scoring the flesh with a cross at the bottom and covering with boiling water for 20 seconds. Peel off the skin and cut the tomatoes into four, then scoop out the seeds.

**2** Blend all the ingredients until smooth. Serve at once, or chill for later use.

✱ Serve *with baby rice cakes or breadsticks, or steamed vegetable sticks.*

# Cheesy polenta "twigs"

Gluten-free polenta or cornmeal can be shaped and baked as a finger food. It freezes well, and so it is worth making a larger batch and keeping for later as it is a wheat-free alternative to breadsticks.

2 mins   5–10 mins   10–12 twigs

## ingredients

¾ cup fine quick-cook **polenta** or **cornmeal**

1½oz (40g) **hard cheese**, such as Cheddar, grated

## method

**1** Preheat the oven to 375°F (190°C).

**2** Place the polenta and ½ cup water in a saucepan and bring to a boil, stirring constantly until the mixture thickens and leaves the sides of the pan. Remove from the heat and stir in the cheese.

**3** When cool enough, break off pieces of the dough and shape into "twigs" 1½–2in (4–5cm) in length and as thick as your finger. Bake for 15 minutes to harden, cool, and store.

\* **Serve** *with dips, or as an alternative to pieces of toast or breadsticks.*

\* **Refrigerate** *in an airtight container for up to 48 hours or freeze when cool.*

# Tofu and avocado dip

Tofu is a bland soy bean curd that is an amazingly good source of calcium, so it is ideal if your baby can't tolerate dairy products. It also provides iron, which the vitamin C-rich tomatoes in the recipe ensure can be easily absorbed.

5 mins   1 min   2 baby and 1 adult portion

## ingredients

1 ripe medium **tomato**
1 ripe small or ½ medium **avocado**

2oz (60g) **silken tofu**
1 tsp **lemon** or **lime juice**

## method

**1** Peel the tomato by scoring the flesh with a cross at the bottom and covering with boiling water for 20 seconds. Peel off the skin and cut the tomato into four, then scoop out the tomato seeds.

**2** Halve the avocado and remove the pit. Scoop out the flesh.

**3** Blend all the ingredients until smooth and serve at once, or chill for up to 24 hours.

\* **Serve** *with steamed vegetables, cooked pasta shapes, or baby breadsticks.*

\* **Best served** *on the day of cooking. Refrigerate in an airtight container for up to 24 hours.*

# Mini lamb and mint balls

These tiny meat balls are a good source of iron and ideal for baby-led weaning. Blend the ingredients together well to eliminate lumpy bits that your baby might struggle to chew.

 5 mins  12–15 mins  15 mini balls

## ingredients

½ small **onion**, roughly chopped

½ small slice of **bread**, torn into a few pieces

5½oz (150g) **ground lamb**

1 tsp chopped **mint**

a little **flour**

1–2 tbsp **vegetable oil**

## method

**1** Process the onion, bread, lamb, and mint until fine and well blended. Check for any large lumps and process again if needed.

**2** Pour the mixture onto a clean cutting board or plate. If the mixture is sticky, add a little flour before dividing into 15 parts. Roll each part into a neat ball.

**3** When they are all prepared, heat the oil in a non-stick frying pan and cook gently over low to medium heat, browning on all sides. Drain on paper towels, cool, and serve 1 or 2 per meal, heated to piping hot, then allowed to cool to body temperature.

Mini lamb and mint balls

✳ **Serve** *with a dip, such as Roasted Mediterranean vegetable dip (see p107) or tzatziki.*

✳ **Refrigerate** *in an airtight container for up to 24 hours or freeze when cool.*

✳ **Variations:** *Use any ground meat, but beef and lamb provide more iron than turkey or chicken. Add garlic or a little grated lemon zest.*

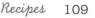

# Baby falafel

An easy food for your self-feeding baby to manage, and a great one to take out and about, baby falafel bites are simple to make and a reasonable source of vegetable-based iron.

 10 mins   15 mins   12 small balls

## ingredients

- 2 tbsp **vegetable oil**, plus extra for frying
- 1 medium **onion**, finely chopped
- 1 **garlic clove**, crushed
- 1 tsp ground **cumin**
- 1 tbsp chopped **cilantro**
- 1 tbsp chopped **parsley**
- 1 x 14oz (400g) can **chickpeas** in water, rinsed and drained
- 1 **egg**, beaten
- **wheat flour** or **gram flour** (chickpea flour), for shaping

## method

**1** Heat the oil in a frying pan and gently cook the onion and garlic until softened, but not browned. Stir in the cumin and fresh herbs and remove from the heat.

**2** Process the chickpeas until smooth.

**3** Add the cooked onion mixture and 1 tablespoon of the egg to the chickpeas and process again, adding more egg if needed, to make a soft but not too sticky mixture. Shape the mixture into loose balls, using flour if it feels too sticky.

**4** Heat 3–4 tablespoons of oil in a frying pan and gently cook the balls in batches for around 10 minutes, turning occasionally, until they are golden brown on all sides. Drain on paper towels and serve warm.

✳ Serve *with Spicy peanut dip (see opposite), natural yogurt, and couscous. (see p102)*

✳ Refrigerate *in an airtight container for up to 48 hours or freeze when cool.*

✳ Variation: *For an older baby or child, mash or process the chickpeas and stir in the cooked onion mixture, rather than processing it all.*

Baby falafel

# Homemade hummus

Using a can of chickpeas is the easiest way to make hummus. If you prefer to soak and boil chickpeas, you'll need around 3½oz (100g) dried beans. Tahini is made from crushed sesame seeds, which are a good source of calcium. You can add the crushed garlic to your portion once you've removed your baby's portion if you prefer.

 5 mins     2 baby and 2–3 adult portions

## ingredients

1 x 14oz (400g) can **chickpeas** in water, rinsed and drained

1 small **garlic clove**, crushed (optional)

1 heaping tbsp **tahini** (sesame seed paste)

1 tbsp **lemon juice**

2 tbsp **extra virgin olive oil**

## method

**1** Blend all the ingredients until smooth. If the mixture is a little stiff, add 1 tablespoon of water at a time to loosen.

**2** Remove your baby's portion and refrigerate the rest. Season your portion to taste.

✽ **Serve** *with pieces of pita bread or vegetables.*
✽ **Refrigerate** *in an airtight container for up to 48 hours.*
✽ **Variations:** *There are many ways to adjust the flavor for yourself and your baby once she is used to this basic version. Try adding a few sun-dried tomatoes or finely grated lemon zest.*

*Homemade hummus*

# Spicy peanut dip

Served warm or at room temperature, this is great with the Mini lamb and mint balls (see p109), or served with vegetable sticks for your baby to dunk. Peanuts are rich in protein and vitamins E and B3. If there are allergies in the family, consult your doctor before giving your baby peanuts.

 5 mins   2 mins  2 baby and 2 adult portions

## ingredients

2 **scallions**, washed, trimmed, and roughly sliced

4 cup **whole milk**, plus extra if needed

½ tsp **garam masala** or **ground cumin**

1 tsp chopped **cilantro**

⅓ cup **smooth peanut butter**, low/no sugar or salt

## method

**1** Place the scallions, milk, garam masala or cumin, and cilantro in a small saucepan and heat gently to soften the onions.

**2** Cool slightly and blend with the peanut butter to make a smooth dip, adding more milk, if needed.

✽ **Serve** *with Mini lamb and mint balls (see p109) or Baby falafel (see opposite).*

# Chicken Provençale

Full of Mediterranean favorites, Chicken Provençale is a great source of vitamin C and is enjoyed by babies and parents alike. It freezes well so make a batch when peppers and zucchini are plentiful to use as your baby grows.

 7–8 mins     20–25 mins     5–6 baby portions or 1 adult and 2 baby portions

Chicken Provençale

## ingredients

1 tbsp **olive oil**
1 small **onion**, finely chopped
4oz (120g) or 1 skinless **chicken thigh fillet**, cut into ¾ in (2cm) pieces
½ **red bell pepper**, quartered and finely chopped

½ medium **zucchini**, quartered lengthwise and sliced
1 x 7oz (200g) can chopped **tomatoes**
6 **basil leaves**, washed and torn
1 tbsp **couscous** or **rice**, cooked

## method

**1** Heat the oil in a non-stick saucepan and gently cook the onion for 2–3 minutes before adding the chicken. Continue to cook for 2–3 minutes until the chicken is lightly cooked on each side.

**2** Stir in the pepper, zucchini, and tomatoes. Stir, cover, and bring to a simmer. Reduce the heat and cook gently for 15–20 minutes, or until the vegetables and chicken are tender.

**3** Add the basil leaves in the last 5 minutes of cooking and, if the mixture is looking dry, add 1 tablespoon of water.

**4** When cooked, remove your baby's portion and adjust the texture. Serve with a tablespoon of couscous or rice mashed into the mixture.

✳ Serve *with pieces of cooked carrot alongside.*

✳ Refrigerate *in an airtight container for up to 48 hours or freeze when cool.*

✳ Variations: *Add a slice or two of eggplant instead of or as well as the zucchini.*

# Fruity chicken

Rich in vitamin A, mango makes a delicious addition to this chicken stew. Using darker thigh meat provides more iron than if you use the whiter breast meat. The raisins also top off the iron quota.

 5 mins     20 mins     6 baby portions or 2 baby and 1 adult portion

## ingredients

1 tbsp **vegetable oil**
1 small **onion**, finely chopped
3½oz (100g) skinless **chicken thigh fillet**, cut into 2cm (¾ in) pieces
½ tsp **ground cumin**
1oz (30g) **raisins**
5½oz (150g) **mango**, cut into cubes (see p131)

## method

**1** Heat the oil in a non-stick saucepan and lightly cook the onion and chicken for 4–5 minutes without browning.

**2** Stir in the cumin, raisins, and ⅔ cup water and bring to a simmer. Stir, reduce the heat, and cook over low heat, checking occasionally, for 10 minutes.

**3** Add the mango cubes and cook for 5–6 minutes, or until very tender.

**4** Cool slightly, remove your baby's portion, and adjust the texture by processing a little before serving.

✳ Serve *with green vegetables.*

✳ Refrigerate *in an airtight container for up to 24 hours or freeze when cool.*

# Chicken and mushroom casserole

Chicken is a good source of protein. As with Fruity chicken (see opposite), using darker thigh meat rather than the white breast supplies more iron. Mushrooms provide iron, too, which the body absorbs more easily than from other plant foods.

⏱ 5 mins    🔥 20–25 mins    🥧 5–6 baby portions or 1–2 baby and 1 adult portions    ❄

## ingredients

1 tbsp **vegetable oil**

5¾oz (160g) skinless **chicken thigh fillets**, cut into ¾–1in (2–3cm) pieces

1 small **zucchini**, sliced

2oz (60g) **button mushrooms**, rinsed and sliced

1 tsp chopped **thyme**

## method

**1** Heat the oil in a non-stick saucepan and cook the chicken until sealed all over. Stir in the zucchini, mushrooms, and thyme with ⅔ cup water.

**2** Bring to a simmer, stir, and cover. Reduce the heat and cook for 15–20 minutes, or until the vegetables are tender and the chicken is cooked through. Remove from the heat and let cool slightly.

**3** If you are eating the casserole too, remove your baby's portion and blend to the necessary texture. Season your portion with black pepper, and if you like, a little salt.

✱ **Serve** *with mashed potatoes or wedges of boiled potatoes, carrots, or squash, and green vegetables.*

✱ **Refrigerate** *in an airtight container for up to 24 hours or freeze in individual labeled containers when cool.*

✱ **Variations:** *You can add 1 small finely chopped onion in step 1.*

# Normandy pork

Made with pork and apples, this dish is bound to be a hit with your baby. For speed use ground pork, but if the oven is on, you can use any stewing pork, cooking it slowly to tenderize it and then processing.

⏱ 5 mins    🔥 30–35 mins    🥧 3–4 baby portions    ❄

## ingredients

1 tbsp **vegetable oil**

½ small **onion**, finely chopped

3½oz (100g) lean **ground pork**

1 medium **apple**, peeled, cored and grated

⅔ cup **apple cider**, plus more if needed

½ tsp chopped **sage**

## method

**1** Heat the oil in a non-stick saucepan and gently cook the onion and pork together, using a spoon to break up the pork. Stir in the apple, juice, and sage and cover.

**2** Simmer gently for 20–25 minutes, or until the mixture is tender, stirring and adding more juice, if needed.

**3** Process to a suitable consistency.

*Normandy pork*

✱ **Serve** *with mashed potatoes or steamed potato pieces and a green vegetable.*

✱ **Refrigerate** *in an airtight container for up to 24 hours or freeze on the day of cooking when cool.*

# Pork with pineapple

Your baby will enjoy this simple sweet and sour style of pork. It uses a can of pineapple pieces in juice, which are softer than fresh pineapple and available cheaply all year round.

 7–8 mins  30 mins  5–6 baby portions or 2 baby and 1 adult portion

## ingredients

1 tbsp **vegetable oil**
5½oz (150g) lean **ground pork**
2 small **celery ribs**, finely chopped
½ small **onion**, finely chopped
1 x 8oz (225g) can of **pineapple** pieces in juice
1 tbsp **tomato paste**
1 tsp **wine vinegar**

## method

**1** Heat the oil in a non-stick saucepan and gently cook the pork, breaking it up with a spoon as it cooks.

**2** Add the celery and onion and continue cooking over medium heat for 2–3 minutes to cook the vegetables.

**3** Drain the pineapple pieces and reserve the juice in a glass measuring cup. Add the pineapple to the saucepan.

**4** Add the sauce and vinegar to the pineapple juice and add water until the cup measures ⅔ cup of liquid. Add to the pan.

**5** Bring to a simmer, stir, cover, and cook gently for 20 minutes, or until the mixture is tender.

**6** Remove your baby's portion and process to a suitable consistency before serving. Season your portion with a little soy sauce, if desired, and serve.

✱ **Serve** *with plain boiled rice and steamed green vegetables as finger food.*
✱ **Refrigerate** *in an airtight container for up to 24 hours or freeze on the day of cooking when cool.*
✱ **Variations:** *Use canned apricots in juice instead of pineapple.*

# Herby lamb with vegetables

This simple recipe uses ground lamb, and if you're making the Mini lamb and mint balls (see p109), it's a great one to cook at the same time, as one 18oz (500g) pack of ground lamb will provide you and your baby with several meals.

 7–8 mins  30–35 mins  4–6 baby and 3 adult portions

## ingredients

12oz (350g) lean **ground lamb**
1 medium **onion**, finely chopped
1 large **carrot**, peeled and finely diced
7oz (200g) **butternut squash**, peeled and finely diced
1 tbsp chopped fresh, or ½ tbsp dried, **mint**
1 tbsp chopped **thyme**
1 tbsp **tomato paste**

## method

**1** Place the lamb and onion in a non-stick saucepan and heat gently, allowing the fat from the lamb to cook the onions. Break the lamb up with a wooden spoon as you continue to cook for 5–7 minutes, or until the lamb is lightly browned.

**2** Add the carrot, squash, herbs, and tomato paste and stir well.

**3** Pour in 1¼ cups water and bring to a simmer. Stir, cover, reduce the heat, and simmer for another 25–30 minutes, or until the vegetables are tender and the lamb is cooked through completely.

**4** Take off the heat and remove your baby's portions—approximately 1 heaping tablespoon of mixture per portion.

**5** Blend your baby's portion to a suitable texture, perhaps reserving some soft pieces of carrot or squash for her to eat with her fingers.

**6** For your portion, adjust the seasoning if you need to, and serve with rice, potatoes, or couscous and a green vegetable.

✱ **Serve** *every tablespoon of lamb and vegetables with 1 heaping tablespoon of cooked rice, blending if necessary, or mashed potato.*
✱ **Refrigerate** *in an airtight container for up to 24 hours or freeze.*

# Baby's first lamb tagine

In this slow-cooked dish, dried fruit and meat provide a sweet iron-rich combination for your baby. Serve with couscous (see p102) for a real Moroccan flavor.

 5 mins   80–90 mins   6 baby portions or 2 baby and 1 adult portion  ❄

## ingredients

5½oz (150g) **lamb**, such as boneless shoulder or cutlet, cut into 2cm (¾in) cubes
1 small **onion**, finely chopped
1 **garlic clove**, crushed
3½oz (100g) **dried fruit**, such as prunes and apricots, halved
½ tsp **ground cumin**
½ tsp **ground coriander**
2 tbsp **tomato paste**

## method

**1** Preheat the oven to 325°F (170°C).

**2** Place all the ingredients with ¾ cup water in a small casserole dish, stir well, cover, and cook in the oven for 1 hour, checking and stirring occasionally, adding more water if necessary.

**3** Return and cook for another 20–30 minutes, or until the lamb is tender. Cool slightly and remove your baby's portion. Process to a suitable consistency and serve.

✱**Serve** *with couscous and cooked pieces of green beans or zucchini.*

✱**Refrigerate** *in an airtight container for up to 24 hours or freeze on the same day when cool.*

✱**Variations:** *Swap half of the dried fruit for raisins.*

# Beef ragu

Beef ragu is a family staple that can be used to make lasagna, served with pasta as a Bolognese sauce, or used as a meaty dip for babies who like to self-feed. Beef is rich in iron and zinc, and choosing lean ground beef will cut down on saturated fats.

 10 mins   35–40 mins   2 baby and 2 adult portions  ❄

## ingredients

1 tbsp **vegetable oil**
½ small **onion**, finely chopped
1 **garlic clove**, crushed
9oz (250g) lean **ground steak**

¼ **red bell pepper**, finely chopped
7oz (200g) can chopped **tomatoes**
2 tbsp **tomato paste**
½ tsp **thyme** or **oregano**

## method

**1** Heat the oil in a non-stick saucepan and gently cook the onion, garlic, and steak, breaking up the meat with a wooden spoon for 5 minutes until the steak is separated. Add the red bell pepper and continue cooking, stirring frequently, until it is soft and the meat has browned.

**2** Add the tomatoes, tomato paste, and herbs with ½ cup water

and bring to a simmer. Stir, cover, and cook for 25–30 minutes, or until the sauce has thickened, adding more water if needed.

**3** Remove from the heat, process to a suitable texture for your baby if needed, and serve at body temperature.

✱**Serve** *with pasta shapes, broccoli florets, and pieces of carrot.*

✱**Refrigerate** *for 48 hours or freeze on day of making when cool.*

✱**Variations:** *You can use lamb or ground pork if you prefer, or even try it with a vegetarian mixture.*

Beef ragu

# Beef and onion casserole

Slowly braised meat becomes tender and easier to eat, which is ideal for babies who are learning to chew. Using beef ensures your baby has a good supply of easily absorbed iron. This is a casserole or stew at its most basic, which you can adapt by adding different vegetables, herbs, or meats.

 10 mins    1½–2 hours    3 baby and 1 adult portion

## ingredients

2 tbsp **vegetable oil**
3½oz (100g) or 1 medium **onion**, finely chopped
14oz (400g) lean braising **steak**, cut into ¾–1in (2–3cm) cubes
9oz (250g) or 2 large **carrots**, peeled and cut into ½in (1cm) thick slices
1 **bay leaf**
1 tbsp **flour** (wheat or cornstarch)

## method

**1** Preheat the oven to 325°F (170°C).

**2** Heat the oil in a flameproof pan and gently cook the onion for 2–3 minutes. Add the beef to the pan and lightly brown on all sides, stirring frequently while browning.

**3** Stir in the carrots and 1¾ cups water, then add the bay leaf. Bring to a simmer, cover, and place in the oven for 1 hour.

**4** Remove from the oven. Mix the flour with 2 tablespoons of water and a little of the cooking juice, and stir this into the casserole.

**5** Cover and return to the oven for 30–45 minutes, or until the beef is very tender and separates easily when cut with a knife.

**6** Remove the bay leaves, take out your baby's portion, and let cool slightly. Blend until the meat is a soft consistency and serve or cool before freezing.

✱ **Serve** *with mashed potatoes and broccoli florets.*

✱ **Refrigerate** *in an airtight container for up to 48 hours or freeze when cool.*

✱ **Variations:** *This recipe can be made with stewing lamb. You can use parsnips, rutabaga, and celeriac instead of, or as well as, the carrots. Remove some carrots before puréeing the meat, and then roughly mash or chop these into the mixture.*

# Beef with prunes

A slowly cooked stew with prunes makes a delicious main course for you and your baby and also freezes well. The addition of a little tomato paste provides vitamin C to help with iron absorption from the beef and prunes.

 5 mins    80–90 mins    6 baby portions or 2 baby and 1 adult portion

## ingredients

7oz (200g) lean braising **steak**, cut into ½–¾in (1–2cm) cubes
1 small **onion**, finely chopped
1¾oz (50g) ready-to-eat **prunes**, halved
¼ tsp **cinnamon** (optional)
1 tbsp **tomato paste**

## method

**1** Preheat the oven to 325°F (170°C).

**2** Place all the ingredients with 1 cup water in a small casserole dish and cover.

**3** Cook in the oven for 1 hour. Check and stir occasionally, adding more water if needed. Return and cook for another 20–30 minutes, or until the beef is tender.

**4** Cool slightly and remove your baby's portion. Process to a suitable consistency and serve.

✱ **Serve** *with mashed potatoes or sweet potato, couscous, and steamed green vegetables.*

✱ **Refrigerate** *in an airtight container for up to 48 hours or freeze when cool.*

# Sweet potatoes with sardines and peas

Canned sardines are an excellent source of many important nutrients including iron, zinc, calcium, and vitamin B12, as well as providing omega 3 fatty acids. Although not always popular, they're an inexpensive "superfood," so it is worth persevering. Buy in water, oil, or tomato paste, and drain well before mashing with a fork or blending.

 5 mins    10–15 mins    3–4 baby portions   ❄

## ingredients

4¼–5½oz (120–150g) or 1 small **sweet potato**, peeled and cubed

1¾oz (50g) **frozen peas**, defrosted

1–2 tbsp **water** or **milk**

1oz (35g) canned **sardines**, drained

## method

**1** Steam the sweet potatoes for 10–12 minutes, let cool a little, and mash.

**2** Steam the peas for 2–3 minutes until hot through, and then purée with the water or milk.

**3** Mash the fish until fine and mix with the pea purée. Stir the mixture into the mashed potato, and serve warm.

❋ Refrigerate *in an airtight container for up to 24 hours or freeze when cool.*

❋ Variations: *Pilchards are just larger sardines, and are equally nutritious.*

# Cheesy mash with fish and peas

A yummy introduction to eating fish. Choose a sustainably sourced white fish such as Alaskan pollock or cod. Even fillets can sometimes have small bones, so check for bones by running a finger over the flesh of the fish.

 10 mins    15 mins    4–6 baby portions    ❄

## ingredients

7oz (200g) **potatoes**, peeled and quartered

2 tsp **monounsaturated spread**, such as olive spread

5in (13cm) small **leek** (only the white part), cut into quarters lengthwise and finely sliced

2oz (60g) skinless **fillet of white fish**

1 **bay leaf**

⅔ cup **whole milk**

1¾oz (50g) **frozen peas**, defrosted

scant 1oz (25g) **hard cheese**, such as Cheddar, grated

## method

**1** Steam the potatoes until tender.

**2** Meanwhile, heat the spread in a non-stick saucepan and gently cook the leek, stirring frequently, until it is just softening.

**3** Add the fish, bay leaf, and milk and bring to a simmer. Cover and poach very gently for 8–10 minutes, or until the fish is opaque and flakes easily. Take off the heat, remove the fish, and discard the bay leaf, saving the milk for blending.

**4** Steam the peas until tender. Mash the potatoes, using some of the saved milk, and stir in the grated cheese.

**5** Mash or roughly blend the fish and peas with a little milk to a suitable consistency. Mix with the cheesy potatoes and serve at once or chill for later use.

❋ Refrigerate *in an airtight container for up to 24 hours or freeze when cool.*

❋ Variations: *You can omit the cheese, or mash 1 tablespoon of cream cheese into the potato instead of the milk and Cheddar.*

*Adjust the texture by keeping the peas and fish as finger food, served with the mashed potatoes.*

# Vegetable finger foods

**Vegetables make great finger foods**, allowing your baby to participate in self-feeding as well as encouraging good dietary habits. Initially, vegetables need to be cooked lightly to soften them, but as your baby gets older, some, such as bell peppers and carrots, can be left raw to provide varied texture and tastes.

## Steaming

Vegetables should be steamed until they are tender when pierced with a sharp knife. After steaming, let cool to room temperature.

### Zucchini

Choose small zucchini, trimming away the ends and cutting into pieces approximately 1in (3cm) in length.

### Pumpkin and squash

**1** Slice off a piece weighing around 3½oz (100g).

**2** Cut away the hard skin and remove any seeds.

**3** Cut into pieces approximately 1in (3cm) in length.

Steamed broccoli florets

### Broccoli and cauliflower

Broccoli and cauliflower should be cut into small florets your baby can hold.

## Green beans

Choose stringless round green beans, and cut into 2–3 pieces depending on their length.

## Carrots, celeriac, parsnips, potatoes, rutabaga, and sweet potatoes

Trim, peel, and cut into pieces before steaming.

## Red bell peppers

Wash, halve, cut away the stalk, and remove the seeds. Cut into strips about ¾in (2cm) wide and 2–2½in (5–6cm) long. Serve raw or roasted (see below)

# Baking or roasting

If the oven is on, it is worth roasting certain vegetables as this increases their natural sweetness.

## method

**1** Preheat the oven to 400°F (200°C).

**2** Carrots, celeriac, parsnips, potatoes, rutabaga, sweet potatoes, squash, pumpkin, and zucchini can be prepared into finger food as above.

**3** Place any of these vegetables on a baking sheet and brush lightly with vegetable oil.

**4** Bake for 20–25 minutes (15–20 minutes for peppers), or until the pieces of vegetables are tender.

**5** Place on paper towels to drain off any excess oil and serve at room temperature.

# Greek baked fish

Dill or small–leaved basil and olive oil provide a traditional Greek feel to this easy fish dish. Use fully ripe tomatoes and a sustainably sourced white fish of your choice. White fish provides essential protein and iodine and B vitamins, while the tomatoes provide vitamin C.

 5–7 mins  15–20 mins  4 baby portions ✳

## ingredients

2 large **plum tomatoes**,
  approximately
  3½oz (100g) each
3½oz (100g) skinless **fish fillet**
1 tsp finely chopped **dill**,
  small-leaved **basil** or **parsley**
1 tbsp **olive oil**

## method

**1** Preheat the oven to 375°F (190°C).

**2** To peel the tomatoes, score a small cross at the bottom of each tomato and place in a bowl. Pour in boiling water and leave for 30 seconds. Remove and peel off the skin. Quarter the tomatoes, remove the seeds, and chop roughly.

**3** Meanwhile, check the fish for bones by running your finger over the flesh.

**4** Place the tomatoes at the bottom of a small flameproof dish and place the fish on top. Sprinkle with the herbs and drizzle with oil.

**5** Cover with a lid or foil and bake for 15–20 minutes, or until the fish flakes easily and is opaque.

**6** Mash or blend the mixture to a suitable texture for your baby and serve immediately, or cool and freeze.

✳ **Serve** with mashed potatoes or sweet potato, Cheesy polenta "twigs" (see p108) or pasta shapes.

✳ **Freeze** in individually labeled portions when cool.

# Italian tomato and tuna mash

Tomatoes, onions, herbs, and garlic are an important part of any Mediterranean diet, and they are combined here with canned tuna for protein, iron, and zinc.

 5 mins  15 mins  5–6 baby portions  ✳

## ingredients

7oz (200g) **potatoes**,
  peeled and quartered
1 tbsp **vegetable oil**
½ small **onion**, finely chopped
1 small **garlic** clove,
  crushed (optional)
7oz (200g) can chopped
  **tomatoes** in juice
¼ tsp dried **oregano**
2oz (60g) can **tuna** in oil
  or water, drained
**milk**, if needed

## method

**1** Steam the potatoes until tender.

**2** Meanwhile, heat the oil in a small saucepan and cook the onion and garlic, if using, until softened.

**3** Stir in the tomatoes and oregano, cover, and cook over low to medium heat for 8–10 minutes, or until the vegetables are tender. Stir in the tuna and heat through.

**4** Mash the potatoes, using a little milk, if needed. Mix the potatoes and tuna together and serve at once.

*Italian tomato and tuna mash*

✳ **Serve** with pieces of steamed green beans, zucchini, or broccoli florets.

✳ **Variations:** For babies who like to feed themselves, serve the sauce with pasta shapes, rather than mashed potato. If your baby needs a smoother mixture, purée the tuna–tomato mixture before adding to the potato.

# Salmon and sweet potato cakes

In this simple recipe, the salmon and sweet potato mixture is formed into little fish cakes, which can be hand held. The mixture can also be used without making it into fish cakes if you and your baby prefer.

 15 mins   20 mins   4 baby and 1 adult portion

## ingredients

9oz (250g) **sweet potatoes**,
  peeled and quartered
7oz (200g) skinless
  **salmon fillet**
1 tbsp **olive oil**
3½oz (100g), or 1 small **leek**,
  washed and finely chopped
½ cup (75g) full-fat
  **Greek yogurt**
zest of ½ **lemon** (optional)
1¾–2½oz (50–75g) **rolled oats**
**vegetable oil**, for cooking

**✳ Serve** *with tzatziki or Roasted Mediterranean vegetable dip (see p107).*

**✳ Refrigerate** *in an airtight container for up to 24 hours or freeze.*

**✳ Variations:** *Use trout fillet. Replace the oats with crushed corn flakes and bake for 20 minutes in the oven at 375°F (190°C).*

## method

**1** Steam the sweet potatoes for 10–15 minutes, or until tender.

**2** Meanwhile, run your finger over the fish to check for and remove bones. Loosely wrap the salmon in foil; place on the potatoes, or, if you have a multi-layered steamer.

**3** Heat the oil in a frying pan; gently cook the leek until soft. When the sweet potatoes are soft, mash with the leek, Greek yogurt, and zest, if using.

**4** Flake the fish and check for bones again, then mash into the sweet potato mixture.

**5** Remove around ¼ of the mixture for your baby. Serve as is, cooling and freezing additional portions, or make into baby fish cakes as below.

**6** Divide the portion into 4 small balls. Coat each ball in rolled oats. Set to one side while you make the 3–4 adult fish cakes with seasoning.

**7** Heat the vegetable oil in a frying pan and cook the fish cakes for 5 minutes on each side until lightly browned. Serve warm.

Salmon and sweet potato cakes

# Creamy salmon and pasta

Encouraging oily fish from an early age will help your baby's brain development because of the omega 3 content. This is a recipe you can do throughout the first few years, adjusting the texture as your baby is more able to chew.

 3 mins   10–12 mins   4–5 baby portions

## ingredients

1¾oz (50g) skinless
  **salmon fillet**
1½oz (40g) **pasta shapes**
1¾oz (50g) small
  **broccoli florets**
2 tbsp full-fat **Greek yogurt**
**whole milk**, as needed

## method

**1** Check the salmon for bones by running your finger over the flesh. Steam or cook in the oven for around 12 minutes at 350°F (180°C) until the fish flakes easily.

**2** Cook the pasta shapes according to the package instructions. In the last 4 minutes, add the broccoli and continue to cook.

**3** Place the salmon in a bowl and flake the fish with a fork, checking again for bones. Stir in the Greek yogurt. When the pasta and broccoli are softened, drain and mix with the salmon.

**4** Process the mixture to an appropriate texture, adding milk as needed. Remove a portion to serve immediately, reheating if necessary. Freeze the remaining portions.

**✳ Refrigerate** *for 24 hours or freeze on the day of cooking.*
**✳ Variations:** *Use cauliflower or zucchini instead of broccoli.*

# Yummy veggie sauce with pasta

As soon as your baby can cope with a few lumps, you can add baby pasta shapes to sauces, or if she prefers, let her hold a soft cooked pasta bow or penne and dip it in the sauce.

 5 mins     20–25 mins     4–5 baby portions

## ingredients

1 tbsp **vegetable oil**

5in (13cm) small **leek** (only the white part), cut into quarters lengthwise and finely sliced

1 small **zucchini**, washed, trimmed, and finely diced

1 **garlic clove**, crushed (optional)

1 x 10½ oz (300g) can chopped **tomatoes** in juice

6 **basil leaves**, washed and roughly torn

### For each portion of sauce:

½–¾oz (15–20g) cooked **pasta shapes**

1 tbsp grated **cheese** to stir into the hot sauce, or 1–2 pieces as finger food

## method

**1** Heat the oil in a non-stick saucepan and gently cook the leek, zucchini, and garlic, if using, for approximately 5 minutes, or until just softened.

**2** Add the tomatoes and basil and bring to a boil. Stir, cover, and simmer for 15–20 minutes, or until the vegetables are soft.

**3** Remove from the heat, let cool a little, blend to an appropriate texture, if needed, and serve with pasta shapes and cheese.

✳ Refrigerate *the sauce in an airtight container for up to 24 hours or freeze in individual labeled containers when cool.*

✳ Variations: *Use a small onion instead of leek, if you prefer.*

# Butternut squash risotto

Any sort of squash or pumpkin will do for this creamy dish. You can use either special risotto rice, or short-grain rice is perfectly fine, too. This is another recipe that you can make for the whole family, taking out a portion for your baby and adjusting the texture of hers.

 10 mins     40–45 mins     1 baby and 2 adult portions

## ingredients

1 tbsp **vegetable oil**

1 medium **onion**, finely chopped

1 **garlic clove**, crushed

10½ oz (300g) **butternut squash**, peeled and cut into ¼in (5mm) cubes

5½oz (150g) **short-grain rice**

1¾–2 cups **salt-free stock** or **water**

1 tbsp chopped **thyme**

### For each baby portion:

1 tsp **Greek yogurt**

### For each adult portion:

grated **Parmesan cheese**

1 tbsp chopped **parsley**

## method

**1** Heat the oil in a non-stick sauté pan and cook the onions over a fairly high heat for 5 minutes until softened and browning. Stir in the garlic and squash and cook over lower heat for 5 minutes, stirring frequently.

**2** Add the rice, ⅔ cup of the stock or water, and thyme. Stir and continue cooking over medium heat for 30–35 minutes, stirring frequently, allowing the liquid to be absorbed before adding more liquid. Continue this until all the stock has been added.

**3** Remove from the heat and let cool slightly. Remove a portion for your baby and blend to a suitable texture, adding the Greek yogurt before serving. Season the remaining risotto and serve with Parmesan cheese and freshly chopped parsley.

✳ Serve *with steamed green beans or asparagus when in season.*

✳ Refrigerate *in an airtight container after cooling for up to 24 hours or freeze when cool. Defrost in the fridge overnight, or cook the frozen risotto in a covered dish at 350°F (180°C) for 20–30 minutes until piping hot, or in the microwave until piping hot.*

✳ Variations: *Use ricotta instead of Greek yogurt and add diced carrots with squash or asparagus stems in the last 10 minutes of cooking.*

# Baby's first vegetable curry

A can of beans in water makes an easy and nutritious base to a vegetable curry. Use a mild curry powder so both you and your baby can enjoy this. If you like, you can season your own portion with anything spicier or hotter once her portion is served.

 5–10 mins      30–35 mins      2 baby and 2 adult portions

## ingredients

2 tbsp **vegetable oil**
1 small **onion**, finely chopped
1 **garlic clove**, crushed
1 tsp mild **curry powder**
    (preferably salt-free)
7oz (200g) **butternut squash**,
    peeled and diced
1 x 7oz (200g) can
    **pinto** or **butter beans**
1 x 7oz (200g) can
    chopped **tomatoes**

For each adult portion:
Seasoning such as:
1 tsp **garam masala**
1 tbsp chopped **cilantro** or **chili
    sauce** to taste

## method

**1** Heat the oil in a saucepan, then add the onion and garlic and cook until lightly browned. Stir in the curry powder and then add the squash, beans, and tomatoes with ⅔ cup water.

**2** Bring to a simmer, then reduce the heat, stir, and cover. Simmer for 20–25 minutes, stirring occasionally, and adding more water if required.

**3** When the squash is tender, remove from the heat and let cool a little. Remove your baby's portion and adjust the texture by mashing or blending before serving. Season your portion and serve.

\* **Serve** *with plain boiled rice, mashed to a suitable texture for your baby, or pieces of naan bread.*

\* **Refrigerate** *in an airtight container for up to 48 hours or freeze in individually labeled portions when cool.*

\* **Variations:** *You can use any type of beans for this recipe. Black-eyed peas provide a great source of folic acid.*
*You can chop instead of mashing at step 3.*

Baby's first vegetable curry

# Ratatouille

Ratatouille is rich in vitamins A and C, and makes use of sun-soaked summer vegetables when they are in season. Make it for your baby from early on, adjusting the texture by mashing at first, then leaving the vegetables as cooked.

 10 mins     50–60 mins     2–3 baby and 2 adult portions

## ingredients

1 tbsp **olive oil**
1 small **onion**, sliced
1 **garlic** clove, crushed
¼ **red** and ¼ **green bell pepper**, diced roughly
2–3 slices **eggplant**, cut into ½in (1cm) cubes

½ small **zucchini**, cut into ½in (1cm) cubes
2 medium **tomatoes**, quartered
1 x 7oz (200g) can chopped **tomatoes** in juice
½ tbsp dried **oregano**

## method

**1** Preheat the oven to 350°F (180°C).

**2** Heat the oil in a flameproof casserole dish and cook the onion and garlic for 3–4 minutes.

**3** Add the peppers, eggplant, and zucchini and stir over medium heat for 5 minutes.

Stir in all the tomatoes and oregano, and place in the oven for 40–45 minutes, or until all the vegetables are tender.

**4** Remove from the oven and cool a little. Mash or blend your baby's portion to an appropriate texture, or select soft pieces for your baby to eat as finger food.

✳ **Serve** *with couscous, rice, or pasta shapes, with a little grated cheese or mashed tofu.*
✳ **Refrigerate** *in an airtight container for up to 24 hours or freeze when cool.*

*Ratatouille*

# Cheesy tomato risotto

A risotto is a good way of introducing your baby to grains of rice. You can cook short-grain or risotto rice until very soft, then mash if needed.

 5 mins     40 mins     6 baby portions or 2 baby and 1 adult portion

## ingredients

1 tbsp **vegetable oil**
1 small **onion**, chopped
2½oz (75g) short-grain or risotto **rice**
1¼–1½ cups salt-free **stock** or **water**
5½oz (150g) **tomatoes**, peeled and seeded
2–3 **basil leaves**, washed and torn
1¾oz (50g) **Cheddar cheese**, grated

## method

**1** Heat the oil in a non-stick saucepan and gently cook the onion until softened. Stir in the rice and ½ cup of stock or water.

**2** Allow the liquid to be absorbed, stirring frequently, before adding more. Continue this until all the stock has been added.

**3** Add the tomatoes and basil, and continue cooking until the rice is completely tender, adding more stock or water if needed.

**4** When the risotto is cooked, stir in the cheese. Remove your baby's portion and adjust the texture if needed. Freeze additional portions.

✳ **Serve** *with steamed broccoli florets or green beans.*
✳ **Refrigerate** *in an airtight container for up to 24 hours or freeze when cool.*

# Cauliflower or broccoli and cheese

A family favorite, this calcium-rich savory dish can be adapted in many ways to suit the whole family. For a younger baby, steam the vegetables until you can simply mash into the sauce, and for an older baby, keep the vegetables a little firmer to encourage chewing. Also try adding a bread crumb and grated cheese topping and baking for a few minutes for a crispy-topped variation.

 5 mins    15 mins    3–4 baby portions

## ingredients

2 tbsp **all-purpose flour**
1 cup **whole milk**
1 rounded tbsp **butter** or **unsaturated spread**
1¾oz (50g) **hard cheese**, such as Cheddar, grated
7oz (200g) **cauliflower** or **broccoli** florets

## method

**1** Place the flour in a saucepan off the heat and use a whisk to stir in the milk. When it is well combined, add the butter.

**2** Heat gently, stirring constantly until the mixture thickens. Remove from the heat and stir in the cheese.

**3** Meanwhile, steam the cauliflower or broccoli until tender. Pour the sauce over the vegetables and mash or process to a suitable consistency before serving.

✳ **Serve** *with pieces of bread and butter and halved cherry tomatoes.*
✳ **Refrigerate** *in an airtight container for up to 24 hours or freeze when cool.*

# Macaroni and cheese

A favorite meal for the whole family, macaroni and cheese is a great source of calcium. Mash or process to the correct consistency for your baby, or serve a little sauce separately and let your baby dip pasta shapes into it. This recipe uses a basic white sauce made with a fairly foolproof all-in-one method.

 10 mins    15 mins    6 baby or 2 baby and 1 adult portion

## ingredients

2 tbsp **all-purpose flour**
1 cup **whole milk**
1 rounded tbsp **butter** or **unsaturated spread**
1¾oz (50g) **hard cheese**, such as Cheddar, grated
2oz (60g) **macaroni** or **pasta shapes**

## method

**1** Place the flour in a saucepan off the heat and use a whisk to stir in the milk. When it is well combined, add the butter.

**2** Heat gently, stirring constantly until the mixture thickens. Remove from the heat and stir in the cheese.

**3** Meanwhile, cook the pasta shapes according to the package instructions. Drain and mix into the cheese sauce.

**4** Process, if needed, to a suitable consistency before serving and freeze additional portions.

✳ **Serve** *with mashed green peas or broccoli florets.*
✳ **Refrigerate** *in an airtight container for up to 48 hours, or freeze in individual portions on the day of cooking.*
✳ **Variations:** *Add 1 tablespoon of tomato paste for a pink sauce. The sauce can also be made in a microwave oven, cooking for bursts of 30 seconds, then stopping to stir.*

# Vegetarian sauté

A nutritious alternative to other soy-based products, quorn is a manufactured "mycoprotein"—a meat-free source of protein—that is high in zinc and iron.

 10 mins  25 mins  4 baby portions

## ingredients

1 tbsp **vegetable oil**
½ small **onion**, finely chopped
1 **garlic** clove, crushed
  (optional)
1 small **carrot**, peeled and
  finely diced
5½oz (150g) **quorn**
1 tbsp **tomato paste**
⅔ cup **water**
1 tbsp chopped **parsley**

## method

**1** Heat the oil in a saucepan and gently cook the onion and garlic for 5 minutes until just softening.

**2** Add the carrot and continue to cook for another minute or so, then stir in the quorn and tomato paste.

**3** Pour in the water and bring the mixture to a boil. Then stir, cover, and simmer for

15 minutes. Check and stir occasionally, adding more water if necessary.

**4** Stir in the parsley and heat through for a minute or two. Cool slightly, then blend to an appropriate consistency for your baby.

**\*** Serve *with mashed potatoes and broccoli florets or green beans.*
**\*** Refrigerate *for up to 24 hours or freeze on day of cooking when cool.*
**\*** Variations: *Add 1–2 tsp ground coriander at stage 2.*
*For extra nutrition and added creaminess, you can stir in smooth peanut butter in step 4.*

# Creamy vegetable korma

Coconut milk provides a creamy texture to this delicious first korma. It contains ground almonds to provide protein, but if you are not introducing nuts, replace with 2 tbsp cooked lentils or beans of your choice, adding more water if required.

 7–8 mins  15–20 mins  4–6 baby portions or 2 baby and 1 adult portion

## ingredients

3–4 small **potatoes**, peeled and
  cut into cubes
1 tbsp **vegetable oil**
1 **onion**, finely chopped
1 **garlic** clove, crushed
1 tsp finely grated fresh **ginger**
1 medium **carrot**, peeled
  and diced
3–4 **broccoli florets**, cut
  into 3–4 pieces
½ tsp **turmeric**
¼ cup **almond flour**
⅔ cup **coconut milk**

## method

**1** Steam the potatoes until tender. Cool slightly.

**2** In a non-stick saucepan, heat the oil and gently cook the onion, garlic, and ginger for 5 minutes, adding a little water if they begin to stick to the pan.

**3** Meanwhile, steam the carrot and broccoli until tender.

**4** Add the turmeric to the onion mixture and stir in all the vegetables. Add the almond flour and coconut milk, stir, and bring to a simmer.

**5** Reduce the heat and continue cooking over low heat for 5 minutes, or until the mixture is well combined and the vegetables soft.

**6** Remove from the heat and cool slightly. Remove your baby's portion to blend or mash to a suitable consistency. If you are eating this yourself, adjust the seasoning to your taste.

**\*** Serve *with a few steamed green beans as finger food.*
**\*** Refrigerate *in an airtight container for up to 24 hours or freeze in individual labeled pots when cool.*

# Garden vegetable risotto

Garden vegetables can mean all sorts of things, but carrots and beans are usually included. Here, edamame beans are used alongside carrots and leek.

 7–8 mins      35–40 mins      8 baby or 2 baby and 1 adult portion

## ingredients

1 tbsp **olive oil**
1¾oz (50g) or ½ small **leek**, quartered lengthwise and finely sliced
1 small **carrot**, peeled and finely diced
2½oz (75g) short-grain or risotto **rice**

1½–1¾ cups salt-free **stock** or **water**
2oz (60g) frozen **edamame**, defrosted
2 tsp chopped **thyme**
1¾oz (50g) **mascarpone cheese**

## method

**1** Heat the oil in a saucepan and gently cook the leek and carrot for 5–6 minutes, or until softened.

**2** Add the rice and ½ cup of stock or water. Allow the liquid to be absorbed, stirring frequently, before adding more. Continue this until all the liquid has been added stirring in the edamame and thyme with the last addition.

**3** Continue cooking until the rice and vegetables are tender. Remove from the heat and stir in the mascarpone.

**4** Remove your baby's portion, mash if necessary before serving, and freeze additional portions. If you are eating the risotto yourself, season with a little black pepper and add some Parmesan cheese.

＊ **Serve** *with additional steamed carrot sticks.*
＊ **Refrigerate** *in an airtight container for up to 24 hours or freeze on the same day when cool.*
＊ **Variations**: *Use petit pois instead of edamame.*

*Garden vegetable risotto*

# Tofu with spinach and rice

Rich in calcium, tofu is a great alternative for babies who can't tolerate dairy products. Mixed with spinach and mashed rice, this dish provides your baby with a nutritious and tasty meal.

 5 mins      10 mins      4–6 baby portions

## ingredients

1 tbsp **vegetable oil**
½ small **onion**, finely chopped
3½oz (100g) frozen chopped **spinach**, defrosted
5½oz (150g) silken **tofu**
pinch of grated **nutmeg**
3½oz (100g) cooked **long-grain white rice**

## method

**1** Heat the oil in a small saucepan and gently cook the onion until soft without browning.

**2** Add the spinach and any defrosting juices and heat for a couple of minutes to combine, stirring constantly.

**3** Remove from the heat, add the tofu, and mash well. Stir well and grate in the nutmeg.

**4** For a younger baby, add the rice and blend the whole mixture. For an older baby, blend the spinach and tofu mixture, if needed, and mix with the rice, mashing as needed, and serve warm.

＊ **Serve** *with steamed cauliflower or halved cherry tomatoes as finger food.*
＊ **Refrigerate** *for up to 24 hours or freeze on day of cooking when cool.*

# Lentil and spinach dhal

Spinach and lentils both provide iron, although plant-based sources are not as well absorbed by the body. Vitamin C helps its absorption, so you could give your baby a drink of well-diluted unsweetened orange juice with this.

 10 mins  25–30 mins  6–8 baby or 2 baby and 2 adult portions

## ingredients

- 1 tbsp **vegetable oil**
- 1 medium **onion**, finely chopped
- 1 **garlic clove**, crushed
- 4½oz (125g) spilt **red lentils**, rinsed
- 2 tsp **ground coriander**
- 2 tsp **ground cumin**
- 1 tbsp **tomato paste**
- 4½oz (125g) frozen **spinach**, thawed

## method

**1** Heat the oil in a non-stick saucepan and cook the onion and garlic for 4–5 minutes until lightly browned. Stir in the lentils, coriander, cumin, and 1¾ cups water, add more if necessary.

**2** Bring to a simmer, stirring occasionally, cover, and reduce the heat. Continue to cook, stirring periodically, and adding more water if the mixture is too dry.

**3** When the lentils are soft, stir in the tomato paste and spinach.

**4** Continue to cook for 5 minutes, or until the dhal is piping hot.

\* **Serve** *with rice, pieces of chapati, or naan bread.*

\* **Refrigerate** *in an airtight container for up to 48 hours or freeze on day of cooking.*

\* **Variations:** *Add 1 tablespoon of freshly chopped coriander in step 3.*

# Coconut lentil dhal

This creamy iron providing dhal is a great dish that can be served early on or later in weaning and childhood as it purées and mashes well, or can be left as it is. As with the Lentil and spinach dhal (see above), the meal could be served with some well-diluted unsweetened orange juice to provide vitamin C to help the absorption of iron, as well as green vegetables.

 5 mins  25 mins  4–6 baby or 2 baby and 1 adult portion

## ingredients

- 1 tbsp **vegetable oil**
- 2oz (60g) or 1 small **onion**, finely chopped
- 1 **garlic clove**, crushed (optional)
- ½ tsp **ground cumin**
- 3½oz (100g) split **red lentils**, rinsed
- ⅔ cup canned **coconut milk**
- 1 tbsp tomato paste

## method

**1** Heat the oil in a non-stick saucepan and cook the onion until soft. Add the garlic, if using.

**2** Stir in the cumin and lentils and cook for 1 minute, stirring, before adding the coconut milk, ¾ cup water, and tomato paste.

**3** Bring to a simmer, stir, cover, and reduce the heat. Simmer for 15 minutes, and if it becomes a little dry, add 1–2 tablespoons of water.

**4** Remove from the heat after 20 minutes, or when the lentils and onions are soft, and let cool a little.

**5** Check the consistency and purée or mash, if needed. Serve your baby's portion, cooling, labeling, and freezing the remainder.

\* **Serve** *with pieces of naan bread or chapati, broccoli florets, or green beans.*

\* **Refrigerate** *in an airtight container for up to 24 hours or freeze.*

\* **Variations:** *Stir in a ½ teaspoon of garam masala after 15 minutes of cooking.*

# Creamy apricot dessert

Apricots provide vitamin A. In summer, use fresh ones to make this easy dessert. Out of season, use canned fruit in juice, draining the juice before blending.

 2 mins      6 mins      1–2 baby portions and 1 adult

## ingredients

9oz (250g) fresh **apricots**
2½oz (75g) **mascarpone cheese**

## method

**1** Wash the apricots, remove the pits, and quarter.

**2** Place in a small saucepan with 2 tablespoons of water, adding more if needed. Bring to a simmer, cover, stir, and cook for 4–5 minutes, until tender.

**3** Cool and blend until smooth. When the mixture has cooled, add the mascarpone and blend again. Spoon into little dishes and refrigerate.

＊**Serve** *with pieces of fresh fruit.*

＊**Refrigerate** *in an airtight container for upto 24 hours*

＊**Variations:** *Use fresh nectarines or peaches instead of apricots.*

# Appley plums

In late summer, when plums are abundant, stew and freeze a few batches to use later in the year as desserts, breakfasts, or to add to crumbles or pies. Depending on the type of plums you use, you may not need much juice for cooking.

 5 mins     2 baby and 2 adult portions

10–15 mins

## ingredients

6 ripe **plums**
⅔ cup **apple cider**

## method

**1** Wash and halve the plums. Remove the pits and cut in half again.

**2** Place in a small saucepan with the apple juice, cover, and simmer gently until soft. Cool and process lightly, if required, before serving.

＊**Serve** *with 1 spoonful of yogurt or cottage cheese.*

＊**Refrigerate** *in an airtight container for up to 48 hours or freeze on day of cooking when cool.*

# Stewed apple and cranberries

Cranberries are a great source of protective plant substances, phenols. As they are sour, sweetened cranberries are used here with apples.

 10–12 mins      10–12 mins      3–4 baby portions

## ingredients

1 medium **apple**, peeled, cored, and chopped into small pieces

1½ tbsp canned **cranberry sauce**

## method

**1** Place the apple pieces in a small saucepan along with the cranberries and ¼ cup of water. Cook over low heat, stirring occasionally until softened.

**2** Remove from the heat and cool. Mash or process to a suitable texture and serve.

＊**Serve** *with yogurt, cottage cheese, or custard.*

＊**Refrigerate** *in an airtight container for up to 48 hours or freeze on the day of cooking when cool.*

＊**Variations:** *Use raisins instead of cranberries. Use the basis of this method to stew other fruits.*

*Stewed apple and cranberries*

# *Fruity* finger foods

**As your baby grows more confident at** grasping objects, you can give her a whole range of fruit to enjoy. Soft fruit is a great first finger food as it is naturally sweet so enjoyed by babies, and can be easily chewed. Always stay with your baby when she is eating, especially if she is having finger foods, which she has a greater risk of choking on.

### Apples and pears

Choose ripe and soft varieties, rather than firm ones.

Wash the fruits and peel with a vegetable peeler.

Quarter the fruits and remove the cores and any seeds. Slice into pieces your baby can easily hold.

### Citrus fruit (oranges, clementines, and satsumas)

Given as whole segments, these can be difficult for a baby to eat because they are juicy and the membranes can cause choking. Prepare these fruits with care.

Remove all the peels and piths. Split the fruits into segments and remove the membranes surrounding each segment, checking for any seeds.

### Blueberries

Wash the berries and dry on paper towels. Cut in half.

### Strawberries

Wash the fruits and remove the stems. Cut in half, or slice if large.

### Grapes

Choose the seedless variety and wash thoroughly. Cut in half, pulling away the skin only if it is tough.

### Kiwi fruit

Peel the fruit and cut in half lengthwise, removing the white core. Slice into pieces your baby can easily hold.

## Stone fruit
### (peaches, plums, apricots, and nectarines)

Choose ripe and tender fruits. Wash the fruits and peel off the skins, or drop the whole fruits in boiling water for 20 seconds first, and then peel.

Halve, remove the pits, and slice into pieces your baby can easily hold.

## Papaya

Choose a small ripe papaya and cut in half.

Scoop out the seeds with a spoon and peel with a sharp knife or peeler.

Slice into pieces your baby can easily hold.

## Avocado

Choose a ripe fruit and cut in half.

Remove the pit, cut in half lengthwise, and peel away the skin. Slice into pieces your baby can easily hold.

## Mango

Choose a ripe mango. Cut away a "cheek" of the mango with a sharp knife, then slice the flesh into a crisscross pattern, cutting down to the peel, but not piercing it.

Push the peel inside out, and cut away the cubes with a knife.

## Bananas

Peel the banana and either cut into a few slices across the banana, or make batons by cutting down the length of the banana, then cutting again into 1–1½in (3–4cm) pieces.

## Raspberries

Wash the fruits and dry on paper towels. The seeds are tiny and can be eaten by your baby.

# Mango ice pops

Mango purée can be quickly frozen to make little ice pops that are perfect for sitting outside on a warm day to eat. Rather than traditional ice pop molds, which are rather large, use small paper cups or ice cube trays and pop in a wooden stick. Be prepared for a mess when your baby eats these: a bib is a must!

 5 mins         6–8 baby ice pops    ❄

## ingredients

7oz (200g) **mango purée**,
   homemade (see p59)
   or store-bought
juice of half a **lemon**

## method

**1** Mix the purée with the lemon juice and pour into 6–8 paper cups or ice cube trays. Pop a wooden stick into the center of each and freeze.

**2** When frozen, place all the molds in a container or bag to prevent frosting.

**3** To serve, remove from the freezer and wait for a minute or so. To check if the ice pop is ready for your baby, touch with your clean finger and make sure it does not stick.

✴ **Variations:** *Try different fruit purées such as apricot (see p60) or peach (see p61) , or mix these with the mango.*

✴ **Take care:** Frozen foods such as ice pops can stick to your child's lips if too cold. Remove from the freezer and allow to warm up a little, checking the ice pop yourself before giving it to your baby.

Mango ice pops

# Mixed berry frozen yogurt

A bag of frozen fruits of the forest contains a range of berries and cherries high in protective polyphenols. For a younger baby, sieve out the seeds; for older babies and children, leave the seeds in as they provide fiber.

 5 mins   4–6 baby portions

### ingredients

3½oz (100g) frozen **mixed berries**, defrosted

2 tsp **confectioners' sugar**, if needed
½ cup full-fat, strained **Greek yogurt**

### method

**1** Purée the fruits until smooth and then pass through a sieve to remove the seeds. If very bitter, stir in 2 teaspoons of confectioners' sugar.

**2** Stir into the yogurt and pour into a plastic container suitable

for the freezer. Cover and freeze until solid.

**3** Remove from the freezer and place in the refrigerator for 10 minutes before serving to make the dessert easier to scoop.

\* Serve *with pieces of fruit or a plain cookie.*
\* *The dessert can be frozen for up to 3 months.*

*Mixed berry frozen yogurt*

# Fruit fool

This uses cornstarch custard instead of the traditional cream. It will work with many different seasonal fruits.

 5 mins  5 mins  2 baby and 1 adult portion

### ingredients

2 tbsp **cornstarch**
2 tbsp **sugar**
½ cup **whole milk**
2 drops **vanilla extract**
4½oz (125g) **stewed fruit**, such as rhubarb, stone fruit,

or berries, sweetened if necessary
½ cup thick **natural yogurt** or **Greek yogurt**

### method

**1** Place the cornstarch and sugar in a saucepan and stir in the milk. Heat gently, stirring continuously until you have a thick sauce. Remove from the heat and stir in the vanilla.

**2** Blend the fruits to make a thick purée and stir into the cooled sauce. Gently mix in the yogurt and pour into little bowls. Cover and chill until required.

\* Serve *with pieces of fruit or a plain cookie.*
\* Refrigerate *for up to 48 hours.*

# Banana custard

A simple creamy dessert most babies (and some adults!) love. Milk contains lactose, a natural sugar, and bananas are also sweet, so although you may be tempted to add sugar, there is no need.

 2 mins 5 mins 2 baby portions

### ingredients

1 tsp instant **vanilla pudding powder**

⅔ cup **whole milk**
sliced **banana** to serve

### method

**1** Mix the pudding powder with 2–3 tablespoons of the milk in a large bowl.

**2** Heat the remaining milk until almost boiling, then pour over the pudding mixture, stirring all the time.

**3** Return to the saucepan and heat, stirring all the time until thickened.

**4** Divide the banana slices between 2 small bowls and pour over the custard over the the top. Let cool.

**5** Keep in the fridge for up to 24 hours, bringing the dessert out of the fridge to warm a little before serving.

\* Refrigerate, *covered; for up to 24 hours.*

# Semolina pudding

Semolina pudding is a simple creamy dessert that your baby will be able to eat easily. You can add stewed or puréed fruit to it, or serve it plain.

 2 mins  15 mins  2–3 baby portions

## ingredients

2 tbsp **semolina**
⅔ cup **whole milk**

1 tsp **sugar**
few drops **vanilla extract**

## method

**1** Place all the ingredients except the vanilla extract in a small saucepan and heat, stirring continuously, until thickened and the grains of semolina are soft.

**2** Add the vanilla extract and cool slightly. Remove your baby's portion and serve warm.

∗ **Serve** with apricot or fruit purée (see pp59–62).
∗ **Refrigerate** in a small airtight container for up to 24 hours.

# Ground rice pudding

This is made by mixing milk, ground rice, and a tiny quantity of sugar: an easy dessert that increases your baby's intake of calcium-rich milk. It's best made fresh, but extra can be refrigerated and microwave heated the next day, ensuring it's well stirred, then cooled.

 2 mins 10 mins 2–3 baby portions

## ingredients

2 tbsp **ground rice**
⅔ cup **whole milk**

1 tsp **sugar**
few drops **vanilla extract**

## method

**1** Place all the ingredients except the vanilla extract in a small saucepan and heat, stirring continuously, until the mixture thickens and the rice is soft.

**2** Add the vanilla extract and cool slightly. Remove your baby's portion and serve warm.

∗ **Serve** with fruit purée (see pp59–62) or mashed fruits.

# Lemony ricotta pudding

Using only three ingredients, this dessert will be enjoyed by babies and parents alike. Think cheesecake, but healthier and simpler!

 5 mins  2 baby portions

## ingredients

2½oz (70g) mild **ricotta cheese**
2 tsp **lemon curd**
1 **digestive biscuit** or **graham cracker**, crushed

## method

**1** Mix the ricotta with the lemon curd and stir in the biscuit or cracker crumbs.

**2** Let stand for a few minutes to soften the crumbs a little, then serve or chill.

∗ **Serve** with fresh fruit such as strawberries, peaches, or pear.
∗ **Refrigerate** in an airtight container for up to 24 hours.

Lemony ricotta pudding

# Rice pudding

A childhood favorite, rice pudding is a calcium-rich, easily digested dessert.

 5 mins      2 hours      2–3 baby and 2 adult portions

## ingredients

2 tbsp **butter**
2 tbsp **sugar**
¼ cup **short-grain rice**

2 cups **whole milk**
2 strips **lemon peel**
1 **bay leaf**
grated **nutmeg**

## method

**1** Preheat the oven to 275°F (140°C). Butter a 1-quart flameproof dish.

**2** Place all the ingredients except the nutmeg in a pan and slowly bring to a simmer, stirring often. Reduce the heat and simmer for 5 minutes. Stir, pour into the greased dish, and place in the oven.

**3** After 30 minutes, remove, stir, and return to the oven. Repeat after another 30 minutes, but remove the bay leaf and lemon peel and top with the grated nutmeg.

**4** Return to the oven for 30–45 minutes, or until the pudding is set but slightly wobbly. Cool before serving.

✱ **Serve** *with stewed apricots or plums (see p129).*
✱ **Refrigerate** *for up to 48 hours. Not suitable for freezing.*
✱ **Variation:** *Add 2 tablespoons of raisins.*

# Fruit with chocolate dipping sauce

This is a cornstarch-thickened chocolatey milk sauce in which your baby will enjoy dunking fingers of fruit, or just fingers!

 5 mins      5 mins     2–3 baby portions

## ingredients

1 tbsp **cornstarch**
1 rounded tbsp **hot cocoa powder**
⅔ cup **whole milk**

2–3 drops **vanilla extract**
assorted **fruits** such as mango, strawberry, and grapes, sliced

## method

**1** Place the cornstarch and cocoa powder in a small saucepan and slowly stir in the milk and vanilla extract.

**2** Heat, stirring continuously, until the sauce thickens.

**3** Pour into 2–3 small bowls, let cool, and serve with fruit pieces for dipping.

✱ **Refrigerate** *the chocolate custard for 48 hours, but cut up the fruits just before serving.*

# Chocolate rice pudding

Worth the wait, this chocolate-rich rice pudding provides essential calcium, and you and your baby will enjoy its creamy flavor.

 5 mins      2 hours      2–3 baby and 2 adult portions

## ingredients

2 tbsp **butter**
2 tbsp **sugar**
¼ cup **short-grain rice**
2 cups **whole milk**
2 tbsp **cocoa powder**

## method

**1** Preheat the oven to 275°F (140°C). Butter a 1-quart flameproof dish.

**2** Place all the ingredients in a saucepan and slowly bring to simmering point, stirring frequently, making sure the cocoa is well absorbed. Reduce the heat and simmer for 5 minutes.

**3** Stir well then pour into the greased dish, and place in the oven. After 30 minutes, remove, stir, and return to the oven. Repeat after another 30 minutes.

**4** Return to the oven for another 30–45 minutes, or until the pudding is just set but slightly wobbly. Let cool a little before serving.

✱ **Serve** *with a few slices of banana.*
✱ **Variation:** *Add 2 tablespoons of raisins.*

# Introducing *Stage 3*

**By the third stage of weaning, which is usually around nine to 12 months,** your baby will be used to having regular meals and be fitting into some family mealtimes. Eating together has many positive benefits for him. Remember, though, that you need to model your behavior for your baby, as he will pick up on your table manners, whether good or bad!

## Progressing through the third stage

In this third stage, the texture of your baby's food changes from being mashed with a few soft lumps and sometimes ground to being ground more of the time or simply chopped. She will also be becoming more confident in drinking from a cup. Keep offering foods that have been tricky to introduce previously rather than write them off. Research shows that the more times your baby is exposed to a food, the more likely she is to eat it.

## What your baby needs now

• Milk is still the core of her diet, and she should have a minimum of 16oz (500ml) day, or 2–3 breastfeeds.

• Your baby's appetite has grown to meet her energy needs as she becomes more mobile. Make sure that energy-rich foods such as full-fat cheese and dairy products feature in her daily diet.

• She should have a wide range of vegetables and continue to eat plenty of fruit.

• Your baby should be able to eat a good range of finger foods now, and you can offer some harder textures, including raw vegetables.

• As your baby approaches one year, there will be more family foods that she will be able to eat. At this point, it's important to remember not to add salt or salted stocks to foods she'll be eating with you. You can remove her portion before adding seasoning for the rest of the family, or add salt at the table for yourself if you need it. As well as being unhealthy for your baby, bear in mind too that although a dish may taste bland or in need of seasoning to you, it won't to her as she doesn't have your experience of taste.

### *Your independent feeder*

As your baby approaches her first birthday, she will have made an amazing amount of progress in many areas of development, and these changes will help her develop the ability to feed herself.

From around eight months, she will also be learning to curl her lip around a sippy cup, and as her coordination improves she will be able to drink water from a cup without a lid at her high chair without too many spills.

Her pincer grip, which develops around nine months, will be getting stronger so she is able to pick up finger foods with her finger and thumb rather than her fist. This also means that she will be able to pick up smaller finger foods such as raisins more easily. As her coordination improves she'll be able to use a spoon to convey food to her mouth, but this takes some practice.

Your baby will be better at chewing, and should be able to cope with lumps in food as well as breaking off chunks of finger food and moving them around her mouth to chew.

## STAGE 3 – at a glance

| | |
|---|---|
| TEXTURE | During the third stage of weaning, the texture of your baby's food changes from being **mashed** with **some soft lumps** and **occasionally ground** to being **ground** more of the time or **chopped**. |
| INTRODUCE | Introduce more flavors into her food, giving her more mild spices and adding herbs so she gets used to stronger tastes. |
| AVOID | Do not give processed meats such as sausages and ham, honey, liver, and whole nuts (see p19). |

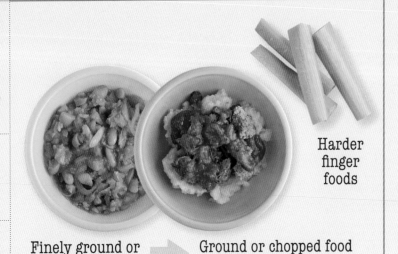

Harder finger foods

Finely ground or chopped food → Ground or chopped food with larger pieces

## Portions for older babies

As your baby's diet becomes more varied and complex, she will eat more finger foods and meals composed of many food groups. The portions guide table for this stage is therefore based on the four main food groups (see p13). Babies, like everyone else, have individual appetites, so the table is just a guide to what the range of intakes may be for this age group.

| FOOD GROUP | WHICH MEAL? | TYPICAL AMOUNT FOR 9–12 MONTH OLD |
|---|---|---|
| Vegetables | Eat at lunch and dinner | 1–2 tablespoons or as finger food |
| Fruits | Any, but at least 2 meals a day | 1–2 tablespoons or as finger food |
| Grains, cereals, potatoes, and pasta | Eat some at every meal | 2–4 tablespoons per meal |
| Meat, poultry, fish, and beans | Eat at 2 meals a day | 1–2 tablespoons for meat, fish, and poultry, per meal<br>2–3 tablespoons if beans or nuts, per meal |
| Milk | Throughout day | 16oz (500ml) formula or 2–3 breastfeeds |
| Dairy – yogurt, cottage cheese | Once or twice a day as dessert or breakfast | 2–4 tbsp dairy foods |
| Finger foods | With meals or occasional snack | Half to one slice bread<br>1–2 baby rice cakes<br>2 strawberries, 5 halved grapes, 1 sliced plum<br>Quarter pear or apple<br>2–3 small vegetable sticks |
| High-fat and high-sugar foods | Not suitable | Not suitable |

# Common sense feeding

**In recent years, much research has been carried out** to see if there is a link between the growth in childhood obesity and the way in which parents approach feeding babies and toddlers. Various studies have come up with theories, but results are conflicting with no conclusive large-scale study. What is clear is that families have individual approaches and attitudes to food, some preferring the routine of set mealtimes from the outset, while others are more relaxed. Your job as a parent is to find an approach that works for you while ensuring that your baby is confident trying new foods that lead him to enjoy a balanced, healthy diet.

## What type of parent are you?

Studies have shown that early childhood preferences help determine food preferences for life. While this is useful information, it also puts a certain amount of pressure on parents. Armed with the knowledge that if their baby eats broccoli at seven months he is more likely to eat it at seven years, many parents feel a big responsibility to get feeding right, perhaps encouraging them to put pressure on their babies during mealtimes that could be counterproductive.

Research has tried to identify whether parents who are more relaxed about weaning bring up babies who are more confident about trying new foods. Or alternatively whether parents who adopt adult healthy eating guidelines themselves mistakenly restrict the food intake of their children. They may cut out certain nutrients, such as fats, that their baby needs to grow and develop healthily.

Whatever your approach to food, being aware of how your baby develops tastes and preferences (see pp48–9) and learns to eat a varied and healthy diet should help you to work out a feeding regime that works for you both. So if you're a parent who likes order, the mess involved in weaning may be challenging. However, recognizing that making a mess is a natural stage in your baby's development that helps him practice his coordination and eventually leads to successful self feeding can help curb your desire to mop up constantly. Putting paper or a splash mat on the floor and a bib on your baby gives you some control over mess, while your baby has the freedom to explore his food.

### Getting it right

Often, anxiety about making sure their baby eats well causes parents to forget common-sense advice:

- Try to be relaxed. If you are stressed about mealtimes, your baby will pick this up. Remind yourself that babies can take several tries before accepting a food, so don't be disheartened if food is rejected. Make eating a social event: talk to your baby, smile, and ensure that mealtimes have positive associations.

- Don't pressure your baby to eat; he'll show you when he is hungry and respond by eating. Swooping spoons and over-persuasion may inadvertently decrease his motivation to eat.

- Banning foods can make them more desirable. Parents who restrict foods can find that when their child is older and goes to other homes, he over-indulges on foods off limits at home. You don't want your child to have cookies each day, but an occasional treat for toddlers is fine.

- Don't expect your baby to eat foods you don't eat. If you never eat your greens, he won't either. Do you need to look at your diet, too?

- Let your baby have some control: the more you restrict or control his food the more likely he is to develop emotional eating behaviors.

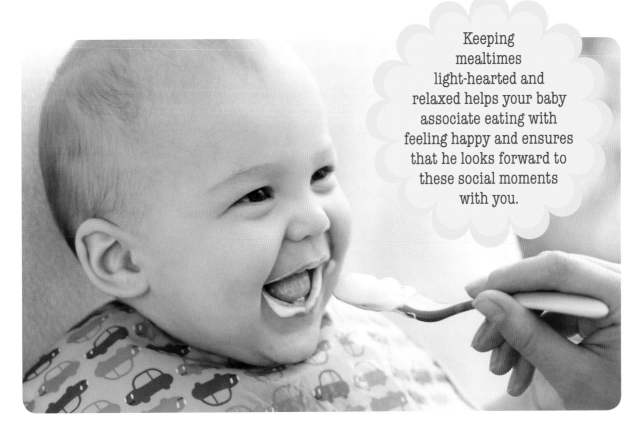

Keeping mealtimes light-hearted and relaxed helps your baby associate eating with feeling happy and ensures that he looks forward to these social moments with you.

## Your baby's temperament

Child psychologists and nutritionists have been looking at whether a baby's temperament has an impact on the way they receive food or are fed, and whether this influences whether they are more likely to become overweight in later childhood.

Some of the types of questions researchers have investigated are:

• Do babies who are difficult to settle become overweight as older children because milk or food is used to comfort them?

• Do some babies respond to parents' over-persuasive attempts to feed them by screaming during feeding or holding food in their mouths, and could this resistance affect growth?

• Are smiley, sociable babies easier to feed because their parents are more relaxed about feeding, or are they more relaxed themselves and this makes weaning easier for their parents?

Different studies have shown a range of answers, but one large study in the UK, called the Gateshead Millenium study, which followed babies from birth up to seven–eight years, showed that there was no evidence that a baby's temperament was likely to lead to him being a greater weight in later childhood. Parents can therefore be reassured that their baby's temperament will not be a barrier to achieving a healthy, varied diet, and that setting up good habits is valuable as these can last into the adult years.

# Eating *together*

**The phrase "family mealtime" may conjure up a picture of a harmonious family** sitting around a table eating healthy food, smiling, and enjoying each other's company. Or it may not! Whether your own childhood experience of mealtimes was a positive or negative one, it is known that children who take part in family meals benefit in a number of ways. It doesn't matter if the meal is a bit chaotic, and manners aren't perfect—it just matters that the family is trying to be together in a shared act.

## Why family meals matter

Many studies have looked at whether eating together as a family makes a difference to family life, and evidence suggests that children who take part in family meals benefit in several ways. When babies and toddlers eat with the family, they are less likely to be overweight and more likely to eat a healthier diet. This is because family meals are more likely to be nutritionally balanced.

There are also social and psychological benefits. Children who eat meals with the family appear to have improved psychological well-being and more positive family interactions. This underpins the fact that mealtimes are not just eating occasions, but social events, too. When family life is busy and hectic, having set times when you eat together provides an opportunity for you to catch up as a family, and establishing family meals early on will benefit your child over the years.

Eating together as a family may also help you to adopt a healthier diet. If you're used to eating frozen meals or processed meats, you may have to review your eating habits when your baby joins you at the table. Like it or not your baby mimics what you do and say, so you can use this opportunity to show her that you eat a wide variety of different healthy meals.

Let your baby watch you prepare her meal and tell her what you are doing to engage her imagination. This way, she'll learn to relate the food in its raw state to the meal that she eats.

### *Setting an example*

Now may be a good time to examine your own feelings about food. If you are a restrictive eater yourself, perhaps you have certain food issues or are dieting, make sure you don't talk about foods being "good" or "bad." Your baby needs to eat a healthy diet that includes energy-dense foods. This may include foods you're avoiding while dieting, such as cheese, oils, or fats, but are important for her to have in her daily diet.

## Making it work

While eating together is the ideal, busy modern lives mean this is often impractical. If you and/or your partner work late, eating together as a family during the week may not always work for you. Rather than feel guilty, think about ways to build in some dedicated family eating occasions:

- Sit down at the table for a meal every Saturday or Sunday, inviting others to join you occasionally. Your baby benefits from these social occasions as she listens to conversation and watches behavior, observing table manners as well as learning language skills.

- Eat lunch with your baby. Rather than tidy up the kitchen while your baby is having lunch, make time to have a sandwich, too. Let her try yours if she wants to.

- If you are cooking for the rest of the family, select some suitable finger foods for your baby to have at the same time as your meal, or adapt the meal so she can have the same. This is often just a case of leaving out the salt, or removing a portion for your baby before adding salt, and chopping or mashing the food. This leads the way to your baby joining in with family mealtimes by one year of age.

- Invite older children to eat at the table; whether these are your own, cousins, or friends, babies love to be with other children, and this makes a simple mealtime into a hugely enjoyable occasion for her. She may want to eat what they are eating, so you might need to adjust the menu. Toddlers can also benefit from being with children who have left the picky stage behind.

- Make food and the family the focus: turn off the television or computer while you eat so your baby isn't distracted.

Eating together and sharing healthy food is a pleasurable experience. And, of course, the occasional treat is fine on special occasions!

# day-by-day meal planner

## Week 1

Salmon and sweet potato cakes

## Monday

### Breakfast
Scrambled egg p99 with toast with melon pieces

### Lunch
Baked potato with salmon, yogurt, and cucumber p176 with steamed green beans
Semolina pudding p134 with mashed kiwi fruit

### Dinner
Beef with prunes p116 with mashed potatoes and steamed broccoli
Exotic fruit salad p191

## Tuesday

### Breakfast
Vanilla and banana smoothie p171 with satsuma pieces

### Lunch
Pea and mint soup p181 with cheese scone p104
Fruit fool p133

### Dinner
Cowboy beans with cornmeal topping p188 with steamed green beans
Blackberry apple cobbler p195

## Wednesday

### Breakfast
Simple muesli p169 with milk and banana slices

### Lunch
Butternut or pumpkin and tomato soup p180 with Egg and sprouts sandwich p175
Greek yogurt with berries

### Dinner
Shepherd's pie (lamb or beef) p185 with roast carrot and pepper fingers
Baked spiced peach p190

## Thursday

### Breakfast
Puffed rice cereal with raisins and milk with mango pieces p131

### Lunch
Ham and pineapple pizza p179 with halved cherry tomatoes
Chocolate rice pudding p135

### Dinner
Salmon and sweet potato cakes p121 with tzatkiki dip and cucumber sticks
Stewed plums p129

## Friday

### Breakfast
Date oatmeal p98
with orange segments

### Lunch
Beef meatballs in tomato sauce p185
with pasta shapes and steamed cauliflower
Mandarin gelatin p192

### Dinner
Bulgur wheat with lamb and eggplant p184
with cucumber sticks
Yogurt and mashed berries

## Saturday

### Breakfast
Mixed berry smoothie p168
Toast and cream cheese p100

### Lunch
Crispy salmon fingers p186 with mashed
potatoes and peas
Crushed canned pineapple with yogurt

### Dinner
Butternut squash risotto p122 with
steamed zucchini fingers
Greek yogurt and fruit purée pp59–62

## Sunday

### Breakfast
Savory muffin p170
with slices of soft pear p130

### Lunch
Macaroni and cheese p125
with halved cherry tomatoes
Mandarins with rice pudding p135

### Dinner
Beef meatballs in tomato sauce p185
with pasta shapes and steamed broccoli
Stewed apple and cranberries p129

Offer your
baby a drink with her
meals—either her usual milk
or water in a sippy cup. If you
wish to give juice, give
unsweetened fruit juice diluted
one part juice to ten parts
water.

*Other ideas this week* Basic oatmeal p98 with banana slices • Toast and peanut butter p101 • Baked beans on toast p173 • Ricotta, tomato, and basil sandwich p174 with carrot sticks • Chicken and pasta with creamy sauce p183 • Chicken Provençale p112 • Baked egg custard p195

# day-by-day meal planner
## Week 2

## Monday

### Breakfast
Bircher muesli p98
with banana slices

### Lunch
Carrot and cilantro soup p181 with
ricotta, tomato, and basil sandwich p174
Yogurt with fruit purée pp59–62

### Dinner
Vegetarian shepherd's pie p189
with steamed broccoli
Baked egg custard p195

## Tuesday

### Breakfast
Banana bread p168 and cream cheese
with clementine segments

### Lunch
Sardines on toast p173 with
cucumber fingers
Appley plums p129

### Dinner
Herby lamb with vegetables p114
with pieces of soft potato and parsnips
Greek yogurt with
apricot purée p60

## Wednesday

### Breakfast
Apricot oatmeal p68
with soft ready-to-eat apricot pieces

### Lunch
Cauliflower cheese p125
with bread and butter
Stewed summer berries p191

### Dinner
Fruity chicken p112 with potato pieces
and steamed green beans
Apple sponge cake p193

## Thursday

### Breakfast
Cinnamon spice pancakes with butter
p99 with soft pear pieces p130

### Lunch
Crêpe with Mexican beans p177
with steamed carrot fingers
Yogurt with mashed blueberries

### Dinner
Salmon and dill risotto p186
with avocado fingers p131
Mandarin ice pop p132

# Friday

### Breakfast
Baked egg with cheese and tomato p172
with clementine pieces

### Lunch
Tuna and avocado sandwich p175
with halved cherry tomatoes
Greek yogurt with fruit purée pp59–62

### Dinner
Chicken mini-burgers p18
with peach chutney p182
and cucumber and pepper fingers
Baked stuffed apple p190

# Saturday

### Breakfast
Teething biscuit p70 with milk and mashed
banana with papaya or melon pieces

### Lunch
Cottage cheese dip p107
with steamed salmon flakes p106 and bread
Stewed apple and cranberries p129

### Dinner
Bulgur wheat with lamb and eggplant p184
with steamed broccoli florets
Yogurt with fruit purée pp59–62

# Sunday

### Breakfast
Baby blueberry pancakes p169
with banana slices

### Lunch
Cheese and tomato tortilla/wrap p177
with cucumber fingers
Mandarins with rice pudding p135

### Dinner
Normandy pork p113 with potato pieces
and steamed green beans
Stewed apple and cranberries p129
with custard

*Other ideas this week* Mango smoothie p171 with toast • Baby falafel p110 with homemade hummus p111 • Leek and potato soup p180 with bread fingers • Creamy avocado pasta p188 with broccoli • Greek baked fish p120 with cooked spinach and potatoes • Apple and pear slices p130

# day-by-day meal planner
## Week 3 2 1

## Monday

Breakfast
Raspberry oatmeal p99
with raspberries

Lunch
Creamy avocado pasta p188
with halved cherry tomatoes
Yogurt with strawberry slices

Dinner
Simple fish pie p187 with
steamed zucchini
Pear and raisin oat crumble p193
and custard

## Tuesday

Breakfast
Carrot muffin p171
with halved grapes

Lunch
Pea and mint soup p181 with
ricotta, tomato, and basil sandwich p174
Pear or peach slices pp130–3

Dinner
Lentil and spinach dhal p128 with rice
and steamed carrots
Greek yogurt with
mashed berries

## Wednesday

Breakfast
Puffed rice cereal with milk
and sliced banana

Lunch
Pesto, tomato, and mozzarella pizza p178
with cucumber and red pepper fingers
Stewed summer berries p191 with ice cream

Dinner
Herby lamb with vegetables p114
with steamed sweet potato fingers
Pear and raisin oat crumble p193
and custard

## Thursday

Breakfast
Scrambled egg p99 and buttered toast
with clementine segments

Lunch
Homemade hummus p111 with pita
bread and red pepper fingers
Yogurt with pitted prunes on side

Dinner
Chicken and pasta with creamy sauce p183
with steamed broccoli and carrots
Ground rice pudding p134
and fruit purée pp59–62

## Friday

### Breakfast
Mango smoothie p171
Toast and cream cheese p100

### Lunch
Simple fish pie p187 with
steamed broccoli and carrots
Melon pieces

### Dinner
Pork with pineapple p114 with
rice and steamed broccoli
Apricot and almond
upside-down cake p194

## Saturday

### Breakfast
Spicy banana toast p100
with apple slices

### Lunch
Tuna and tomato pizza p179 with
carrot and red pepper
Stewed summer berries p191

### Dinner
Shepherd's pie with beef p185
with steamed cauliflower florets
Baked spiced peach p190

## Sunday

### Breakfast
Corn and tomato fritter p172
with mixed berry smoothie p168

### Lunch
Pineapple and cheese on toast p173
with cucumber and halved cherry tomatoes
Pear or plum slices pp130–3

### Dinner
Crispy salmon fingers p186 with mashed
potatoes, cucumber, and avocado dip p105
Passion fruit and mango dessert p91

Greek yogurt

*Other ideas this week* Teething biscuit with milk p70 with fruit • Tuna and avocado sandwich p175 with steamed zucchini • Fruity couscous with peanut sauce p189 • Bulgur wheat with currants and chickpeas p187• Beef ragu p115 with pasta and broccoli • Semolina pudding p134 with fruit

# day-by-day meal planner

## Week 4 3 2 1

## Monday

### Breakfast
Banana bread p168 with cream cheese with papaya or soft pear slices pp130–3

### Lunch
Pineapple and cheese on toast p173 with red pepper fingers
Stewed apple and cranberries p129

### Dinner
Chicken Provençale p112 with soft cooked potato and zucchini pieces
Baked egg custard p195 with berries

## Tuesday

### Breakfast
Baked egg with cheese and tomato p172 with halved grapes

### Lunch
Baked beans on toast p173
Stewed summer berries p191

### Dinner
Vegetarian sauté p126 with pasta shapes and steamed broccoli
Pear and raisin oat crumble p193

## Wednesday

### Breakfast
Mixed berry smoothie p168
Toast and cream cheese p100

### Lunch
Cauliflower cheese p125 with bread and butter and halved cherry tomatoes
Melon or pear pieces p130

### Dinner
Crispy salmon fingers p186 with homemade tomato salsa p182, mashed potatoes, and steamed green beans
Yogurt and kiwi slices

## Thursday

### Breakfast
Date oatmeal p98 with banana slices

### Lunch
Turkey and red pepper patties p184 with homemade tomato salsa p182, bread and butter, and cucumber fingers
Semolina pudding p134 and mandarins

### Dinner
Baby's first lamb tagine p115 with couscous p102, steamed carrots, and broccoli
Passion fruit and mango dessert p191

## Friday

### Breakfast
Teething biscuit with milk p70 with
apricot purée p60
Kiwi slices

### Lunch
Greek baked fish p120 with soft
potato and broccoli pieces
Apple sponge cake p193
with custard

### Dinner
Creamy vegetable korma p126
with rice and strips of naan bread
Mixed berry frozen yogurt p133

## Saturday

### Breakfast
Baked eggs with cheese and
tomato p172 with clementine segments

### Lunch
Mushroom and onion pizza p178
with carrot and pepper sticks
Bread and butter pudding p194 with raisins

### Dinner
Salmon and dill risotto p186
with steamed broccoli
Whole or mashed berries

## Sunday

### Breakfast
Simple muesli p169 with two soft
ready-to-eat apricots

### Lunch
Baked potatoes with spicy chicken
and vegetables p176
with cucumber fingers
Banana custard p133

### Dinner
Beef and onion casserole p116
with potatoes and broccoli
Stewed apple and cranberries
p129 and custard

*Other ideas this week* Baby blueberry pancakes p169 • Pea and mint soup p181 with pita • Hard-boiled egg with buttered toast p69 Garden vegetable risotto p127 • Beef meatballs in tomato sauce p185 with broccoli • Apricot and almond upside-down cake p194

# day-by-day meal planner
## Week
### 6 5 4 3 2 1

## Monday

### Breakfast
Baked egg with cheese and tomato p172 with canned peach slices

### Lunch
Sardines on toast p173
with red pepper/cucumber sticks
Greek yogurt with stewed fruit p129

### Dinner
Beef meatballs in tomato sauce p185
with pasta shapes and
steamed broccoli
Fruit and custard

## Tuesday

### Breakfast
Bircher muesli p98
with dried apple slices

### Lunch
Macaroni and cheese p125
with steamed broccoli/carrots
Apricot and almond upside-down
cake p194

### Dinner
Salmon and dill risotto p186
with avocado fingers
Mango ice pop p132

## Wednesday

### Breakfast
Spicy peach breakfast p96
with banana slices

### Lunch
Cowboy beans with cornmeal topping
p188 with steamed carrots
Greek yogurt with strawberry slices

### Dinner
Normandy pork p113 with couscous p102,
steamed cauliflower, and green beans
Berries with chocolate dipping
sauce p135

## Thursday

### Breakfast
Baby blueberry pancakes p169 with cream cheese
Mango or peach pieces p131

### Lunch
Baked potato with spicy chicken and vegetables
p176 with red pepper and cucumber fingers
Yogurt with mashed kiwi

### Dinner
Sweet potatoes with sardines and peas p117
with steamed carrots and green beans
Stewed summer berries p191
or pear pieces p130

# Friday

### Breakfast
Teething biscuit with milk p70 and raisins
with pear slices p130

### Lunch
Coconut lentil dhal p128 with rice,
pita bread, and green beans
Banana custard p133

### Dinner
Fruity chicken p112 with mashed corn,
steamed sweet potato pieces, and broccoli
Pear or apple pieces p130

# Saturday

### Breakfast
Scrambled egg p99 with buttered toast
p69 with clementine segments

### Lunch
Tuna and avocado sandwich p175
with cucumber fingers
Yogurt with sliced fruit

### Dinner
Shepherd's pie (beef or lamb) p185
with steamed sugar snaps
Baked stuffed apple p190

# Sunday

### Breakfast
Mango smoothie p171
with carrot muffins p171

### Lunch
Leek and potato soup p180
with cheese scone p104
Sliced banana or berries

### Dinner
Greek baked fish p120 with mashed
potato, broccoli, and peas
Chocolate rice pudding p135

*Other ideas this week* Date oatmeal p98 with clementines • Carrot and cilantro soup p180 with bread and butter • Fruity couscous with peanut sauce p189 • Vegetarian shepherd's pie p189 • Simple fish pie p187 with steamed green beans • Exotic fruit salad p191

# day-by-day meal planner
## Week 7 6 5

## Monday

### Breakfast
Raspberry oatmeal p99
with banana slices

### Lunch
Cheesy tomato risotto p124
with pepper and carrot sticks
Creamy apricot dessert p129

### Dinner
Simple fish pie p187
with steamed broccoli
Pear and raisin oat crumble
p193 with custard

## Tuesday

### Breakfast
Banana bread p168
with cream cheese
Mixed berry smoothie p168

### Lunch
Baked potato or wrap with
Mexican beans p177 with cucumber
Fruit fool p133

### Dinner
Beef meatballs in tomato sauce
p185 with pasta shapes and
steamed broccoli
Baked spiced peach p190
with yogurt

## Wednesday

### Breakfast
Buttered brioche slices with yogurt
and strawberry slices

### Lunch
Italian tomato and tuna mash p120 with
cooked spinach
Orange segments with Greek yogurt

### Dinner
Chicken mini-burgers with fruity sauce p183
with steamed broccoli
Stewed apple and cranberries p129
with custard

## Thursday

### Breakfast
Simple muesli p169 with milk or yogurt
with papaya or mango slices p131

### Lunch
Vegetarian sauté p126 with steamed
sweet potato and green beans
Mandarin gelatin p192

### Dinner
Shepherd's pie p185
with steamed parsnip or rutabaga
Mixed berry smoothie p168

## Friday

Breakfast
Puffed rice cereal with milk
with soft dried prunes

Lunch
Beef ragu p115 with pasta shapes and
steamed snow peas
Fruit fool p133

Dinner
Butternut squash risotto p122 with cooked
spinach and steamed zucchini fingers
Blackberry apple cobbler p195
with yogurt

## Saturday

Breakfast
Cinnamon spice pancakes p99 with
butter and strawberry slices

Lunch
Scrambled egg p99 on English muffin
with carrot or pepper sticks
Semolina pudding p134 with apricot
purée p60

Dinner
Pork with pineapple p114 and rice
with steamed celery and green beans
Mixed berry frozen
yogurt p133

## Sunday

Breakfast
Stewed apple and raisins p129 with toast
fingers with hard-boiled egg wedges p69

Lunch
Vegetarian shepherd's pie p189
with steamed cauliflower
Yogurt with raspberries

Dinner
Creamy salmon and pasta p121
with steamed sugar snaps
Crêpes p192 with
stewed fruit p129

*Other ideas this week* Baby blueberry pancakes p169 • Corn and tomato fritters p172 • Pea and mint soup p181 • Chicken and pasta with creamy sauce p183 with broccoli • Cowboy beans with cornmeal topping p188 • Stewed summer berries p191

# day-by-day meal planner
## Week 8  7 6 5

## Monday

### Breakfast
Toast and cream cheese p100
with orange segments

### Lunch
Ham and pineapple pizza p179 with
pepper sticks
Stewed summer berries p191 and yogurt

### Dinner
Creamy vegetable korma p126
with strips of naan bread
Rice pudding p135
with dried fruit

## Tuesday

### Breakfast
Simple muesli p169
with banana slices

### Lunch
Salmon and sweet potato cakes p121
with tzatziki and cucumber sticks
Banana custard p133

### Dinner
Chicken and pasta with creamy sauce
p183 with broccoli
Rice pudding p135 with
canned mandarins

## Wednesday

### Breakfast
Teething biscuit with milk p70
with soft dried apple pieces

### Lunch
Bulgur wheat with currants and chickpeas p187
with tomato quarters
Banana with chocolate dipping sauce p135

### Dinner
Beef ragu p115 with pasta shapes and
mashed peas
Passion fruit and
mango dessert p191

## Thursday

### Breakfast
Toast with hard-boiled egg wedges p69
Kiwi slices

### Lunch
Creamy salmon and pasta p121
with steamed green beans
Yogurt with stewed summer stone fruits
p129

### Dinner
Herby lamb with vegetables p114
with steamed potato pieces
Bread and butter pudding p194

# Friday

### Breakfast
Yogurt with mashed berries
with bread and butter fingers

### Lunch
Macaroni and cheese p125
with halved cherry tomatoes
Mango ice pop p132

### Dinner
Salmon and dill risotto p186
with steamed sugar snaps
Appley plums p129

# Saturday

### Breakfast
Scrambled egg p99 with buttered
toast p69 with orange segments

### Lunch
Carrot and cilantro soup p181
with savory muffins p170
Rice pudding p135 with dried fruit

### Dinner
Turkey and red pepper patties
p184 with peach chutney p182
and steamed green beans
Creamy apricot dessert p129

# Sunday

### Breakfast
Puffed rice cereal with milk
and banana slices

### Lunch
Mini lamb and mint balls p109
with avocado dip p105 and
peppers
Mandarin gelatin p192

### Dinner
Garden vegetable risotto p127
Stewed plums p129

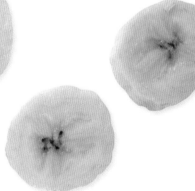

*Other ideas this week* Toast and peanut butter p101 and mango smoothie p171 • Broccoli cheese p125 with bread and butter • Ricotta, tomato, and basil sandwich p174 with carrot sticks • Chicken mini-burgers with fruity sauce p183 with green beans and bread • Yogurt and fruit

# day-by-day meal planner

## Week 9

## Monday

Breakfast
Mixed berry smoothie p168
with baby blueberry pancakes p169

Lunch
Cheesy tomato risotto p124
with steamed carrots
Stewed summer berries p191 and yogurt

Dinner
Chicken mini-burgers with fruity sauce
p183 with sweet potato and broccoli
Baked stuffed apple p190
and custard

## Tuesday

Breakfast
Spicy banana toast p100 with sliced
strawberries or whole raspberries

Lunch
Mini lamb and mint balls p109 with
couscous p102, tzatziki, and cucumber
Segments of clementine or peach slices

Dinner
Vegetarian shepherd's pie p189 with
peas and steamed carrots
Exotic fruit salad p191

## Wednesday

Breakfast
Puffed rice cereal with raisins
and milk and pear slices p130

Lunch
Baked beans on toast p173
Yogurt with berries

Dinner
Simple fish pie p187 with
corn and steamed sugar
snaps
Baked egg custard p195

## Thursday

Breakfast
Simple muesli p169 with milk
and dried apple slices

Lunch
Creamy avocado pasta p188
with steamed broccoli fingers
Mango ice pop p132

Dinner
Vegetarian sauté p126
with potato and parsnip or
rutabaga
Bread and butter pudding p194
with banana slices

# Friday

### Breakfast
Scrambled egg p99 with buttered toast p69
and dried apricots

### Lunch
Pineapple and cheese on toast p173
with cucumber fingers
Semolina pudding p134 with mashed berries

### Dinner
Beef ragu p115 with pasta shapes
and steamed broccoli
Pear and raisin oat crumble p193

# Saturday

### Breakfast
Banana bread p168 with
cream cheese and halved grapes

### Lunch
Sardines on toast p173
with red pepper and carrot sticks
Ground rice pudding p134
with mandarins

### Dinner
Cauliflower or broccoli cheese p125
with bread and butter
Clementine or peach slices

# Sunday

### Breakfast
Raspberry oatmeal p99
with strawberry or mango slices

### Lunch
Butternut or pumpkin and tomato soup
p180 with bread and butter fingers and
cubes of cheese
Mango smoothie p171

### Dinner
Fruity chicken p112 with couscous p102
and steamed green beans
Pear and raisin oat crumble p193
with ice cream

Banana bread

*Other ideas this week* Teething biscuit with milk p70 and fruit • Pea and mint soup p181 with toast fingers • Mushroom and onion pizza p178 • Normandy pork p113 with potatoes and green beans • Crispy salmon fingers p186 with broccoli and potatoes • Chocolate rice pudding p135

# day-by-day meal planner

# Week 10

## Monday

### Breakfast
Scrambled egg p99 with buttered toast p69 and orange segments

### Lunch
Butternut or pumpkin and tomato soup p180 with tuna and avocado sandwich p175
Greek yogurt with kiwi slices

### Dinner
Vegetarian shepherd's pie p189 with steamed green beans
Baked spiced peach p190 with ice cream

## Tuesday

### Breakfast
Vanilla and banana smoothie p171 with corn and tomato fritter p172

### Lunch
Baby falafel p110 with mashed potatoes, cooked spinach, and homemade tomato salsa p182
Greek yogurt

### Dinner
Greek baked fish p120 with potato pieces and green beans
Chocolate rice pudding p135

## Wednesday

### Breakfast
Spicy plum and banana breakfast p96 with pear slices p130

### Lunch
Tortilla with Mexican beans p177 with cucumber fingers
Mixed berry frozen yogurt p133

### Dinner
Bulgur wheat with lamb and eggplant p184 with steamed broccoli or zucchini
Stewed apple and cranberries p129

## Thursday

### Breakfast
Bircher muesli p98 with strawberry or mango slices p131

### Lunch
Ham and pineapple pizza p179 with pepper and carrot fingers
Pear or apple slices p130

### Dinner
Beef meatballs in tomato sauce p185 with rice and steamed sugar snaps
Crêpes p192 with any fruit

## Friday

Breakfast
Carrot muffin p171
with blueberries

Lunch
Salmon and dill risotto p186
with peas mixed in
Mango ice pop p132

Dinner
Pork with pineapple p114 with rice,
peas, and steamed carrots
Canned pineapple chunks

## Saturday

Breakfast
Puffed rice cereal with raisins, milk,
and banana slices

Lunch
Scrambled egg p99 with buttered toast
p169 and halved cherry tomatoes
Greek yogurt with stewed apricots p129

Dinner
Shepherd's pie (with beef or lamb) p185
with steamed parsnip and zucchini
Fruit fool p133

## Sunday

Breakfast
Baked eggs with cheese and tomato
p172 with bread and butter fingers

Lunch
Pea and mint soup p181
with savory muffins p170
Fruit fool p133

Dinner
Chicken Provençale p112
with steamed potato and
broccoli pieces
Banana custard p133

*Other ideas this week* Greek yogurt with banana slices • Hard-boiled egg with buttered toast p69 • Crêpe with cheese and tomato p177 • Simple fish pie p187 with green beans • Normandy pork p113 with potatoes and broccoli • Passion fruit and mango dessert p191

# day-by-day meal planner
# Week 11 10 9

## Monday

### Breakfast
Bircher muesli p98
with blueberries or mango cubes

### Lunch
Mini lamb and mint balls p109 with
couscous p102 and avocado dip p105
Banana custard p133

### Dinner
Fruity chicken p112 with potato,
steamed cauliflower, and broccoli
Chocolate rice pudding p135

## Tuesday

### Breakfast
French toast p98 with currant bun
and dried apricots, halved

### Lunch
Beef with prunes p116 with sweet potato mash
and steamed broccoli
Stewed summer berries p191 and yogurt

### Dinner
Bulgur wheat with currants
and chickpeas p187 with soft cooked
carrot and rutabaga
Bread and butter
pudding p194

## Wednesday

### Breakfast
Puffed rice cereal with raisins, milk, and
clementine segments

### Lunch
Crêpes p192 with salmon, yogurt, and
cucumber p176 with pepper fingers
Yogurt with berries

### Dinner
Chicken and mushroom
casserole p113 with rice,
steamed broccoli, and carrots
Baked egg custard p195

## Thursday

### Breakfast
Buttered brioche slices, yogurt,
and raspberries or strawberries

### Lunch
Vegetarian sauté p126
with pasta and steamed broccoli
Lemony ricotta pudding p134

### Dinner
Turkey and red pepper patties
p184 with couscous p102, peach
chutney p182, and tomatoes
Exotic fruit salad p191

# Friday

Breakfast
Date oatmeal p98
with kiwi slices

Lunch
Leek and potato soup p180
with egg and sprouts sandwich p175
Melon or mango cubes

Dinner
Shepherd's pie with beef p185 and peas
Baked spiced peach p190
with ice cream

# Saturday

Breakfast
Apple yogurt breakfast with
dried prunes, halved

Lunch
Crêpe p192 slices with spicy
chicken and vegetables p176
Stewed plums p129 and custard

Dinner
Salmon and dill risotto p186 with
steamed green beans and broccoli
Pear and raisin oat crumble p193
with ice cream

# Sunday

Breakfast
Scrambled egg p99 with buttered toast p69
Mango smoothie p171

Lunch
Pesto, tomato, and mozzarella pizza p178
with cucumber wedges
Pear or plum slices pp130–3

Dinner
Coconut lentil dhal p128 with naan bread and
steamed green beans
Exotic fruit salad p191

Mini lamb and mint balls

**Other ideas this week** Basic oatmeal p98 with fruit • Ricotta, tomato, and basil sandwich p174 with carrot and pepper sticks • Baked beans on toast p173 • Greek baked fish p120 with potatoes and cooked spinach • Creamy avocado pasta p188 with broccoli • Fruit fool p133

# day-by-day meal planner
## Week 12 11 10 9 8 7

## Monday

### Breakfast
Simple muesli p169
with dried apricots

### Lunch
Crispy salmon fingers p186
with bread and butter, homemade tomato
salsa p182, and cucumber fingers
Greek yogurt with stewed fruit p129

### Dinner
Shepherd's pie (lamb or beef) p185
with steamed sugar snaps and carrots
Lemony ricotta
pudding p134

## Tuesday

### Breakfast
Puffed rice cereal with raisins, milk,
and berries

### Lunch
Pineapple and cheese on toast p173 with
halved cherry tomatoes and cucumber
Banana custard p133

### Dinner
Creamy vegetable korma p126 with rice
and steamed broccoli
Mandarin gelatin p192

## Wednesday

### Breakfast
French toast p98 with currant bun
and orange segments

### Lunch
Scrambled egg p99 with halved cherry
tomatoes and bread and butter
Yogurt with berries

### Dinner
Normandy pork p113 with potato mashed
with corn and steamed rutabaga/parsnip
Rice pudding p135

## Thursday

### Breakfast
Vanilla and banana smoothie p171
with carrot muffin p171

### Lunch
Sardines on toast p173
with cucumber fingers
Banana with chocolate dipping sauce p135

### Dinner
Fruity chicken p112 with mashed
carrot and rutabaga and pasta shapes
Yogurt

## Friday

### Breakfast
Cornflakes with milk
and banana slices

### Lunch
Baby falafel p110 with tzatziki, pita bread
strips, and tomato slices
Mixed berry frozen yogurt p133

### Dinner
Butternut squash risotto p122
with steamed green beans
Crêpes p192 with
stewed fruit p129

## Saturday

### Breakfast
Bircher muesli p98
with chopped prunes or figs

### Lunch
Beef ragu p115 with cooked spinach and
pasta shapes
Exotic fruit salad p191

### Dinner
Simple fish pie p187 with steamed sugar snaps
Stewed summer berries p191
and yogurt

## Sunday

### Breakfast
French toast p98 with currant bun
and clementine segments

### Lunch
Cowboy beans with cornmeal topping p188
with steamed broccoli
Chocolate rice pudding p135

### Dinner
Herby lamb with vegetables p114
and added peas with potato wedges
Baked stuffed apple p190 and custard

**Other ideas this week** Teething biscuit with milk p70 with apricot purée p60 • Tuna and avocado sandwich p175 with red bell peppers • Carrot and cilantro soup p181 with bread and butter • Beef ragu p115 with pasta and broccoli • Salmon and dill risotto p186 with green beans • Baked egg custard p195

# day-by-day meal planner
## Week 13

## Monday

### Breakfast
Spicy banana toast p100 with pear or apple slices p130

### Lunch
Tuna and tomato pizza p179 with carrot/pepper sticks
Mandarin gelatin p192

### Dinner
Shepherd's pie with beef p185 with steamed carrots and sugar snaps
Blackberry apple cobbler p195

## Tuesday

### Breakfast
Baby blueberry pancakes p169 with butter and clementine segments

### Lunch
White flaked fish p106, avocado dip p105, pita strips, and cherry tomato pieces
Yogurt with berries

### Dinner
Pork with pineapple p114 with rice, carrots, and peas
Bread and butter pudding p194

## Wednesday

### Breakfast
Banana bread p168 with cream cheese and berries

### Lunch
Egg and sprouts sandwich p175 with halved grapes and clementine segments
Mixed berry smoothie p168

### Dinner
Fruity chicken p112 with mashed sweet potato, steamed broccoli, and sugar snaps
Rice pudding p135 with kiwi slices

## Thursday

### Breakfast
Bircher muesli p98 with orange segments

### Lunch
Cheesy tomato risotto p124 with steamed broccoli and carrots
Dried apricots

### Dinner
Beef ragu p115 with pasta shapes, spinach, and steamed carrots
Stewed summer berries p191 and yogurt

# Friday

### Breakfast
Scrambled egg p99 with buttered
toast fingers p69 and berries

### Lunch
Tortilla with Mexican beans p177
with cucumber pieces
Apple sponge cake p193

### Dinner
Turkey and red pepper patties p184,
roasted Mediterranean vegetable dip
p107, and bread and butter
Exotic fruit salad p191

# Saturday

### Breakfast
Mixed berry smoothie p168
with savory muffins p170

### Lunch
Tuna and avocado sandwich p175
with cherry tomato pieces
Greek yogurt with stewed fruit p129

### Dinner
Vegetarian shepherd's pie p189
with steamed green vegetables
Pear and raisin oat
crumble p193 with ice cream

# Sunday

### Breakfast
Simple muesli p169
with strawberry or mango slices

### Lunch
Carrot and cilantro soup p181
with cheese scone p104
Banana slices with ice cream

### Dinner
Beef meatballs in tomato sauce
p185 with mashed peas and potato
Apricot and almond upside-down
cake p194

Mexican beans

*Other ideas this week* French toast with fruit p98 • Baked potato with cheese and tomato p177 • Ham and pineapple pizza p179 • Crispy salmon fingers p186 with mashed peas • Creamy avocado pasta p188 with broccoli • Baked stuffed apple p190

Banana bread

# Banana bread

Many banana bread recipes are really cakes, but this one doesn't use sugar, relying instead on the sweetness of the ripe banana.

 5 mins    30–35 mins    8 baby portions

## ingredients

¼ cup **vegetable oil**, plus extra for greasing
2 large ripe **bananas** or 7oz (200g) after peeling
2 large **eggs**

1 tsp **vanilla extract**
1 cup **all-purpose flour**
1 cup **whole wheat flour**
2 tsp **baking powder**

## method

**1** Preheat the oven to 375°F (190°C). Lightly oil a 9 x 5in (23 x 13cm) loaf pan.

**2** Mash the bananas until smooth and place in a mixing bowl. Stir in the oil, eggs, and vanilla extract.

**3** Sift the flours and baking powder, adding back any that stays in the sifter.

**4** Stir the dry ingredients into the wet mixture and beat together until smooth. Pour or spoon into the prepared pan and bake for 30–35 minutes, or until risen and lightly browned.

**5** Cool on a wire rack, then slice and store.

\* Serve *with cream cheese, butter, or spread.*
\* Refrigerate *or freeze on the day of making when cooled.*

# Mixed berry smoothie

You can use almost any kind of berry for this delicious smoothie, so choose whichever fruits you and your baby particularly enjoy and are in season. In winter, you can use frozen berries, either individually, or look out for packages of frozen mixed berries.

 5 mins       1–2 baby portions

## ingredients

3½oz (100g) **berries**, such as **blueberries, strawberries, cherries,** or **raspberries**
⅓ cup **natural yogurt**

## method

**1** If using fresh fruits, remove the stems and wipe with damp paper towel.

**2** Process the ingredients until smooth.

**3** Serve half of it immediately in a cup and chill the remainder.

\* Serve *for breakfast.*
\* Refrigerate *in an airtight container for 24 hours.*

# Baby blueberry pancakes

Blueberry pancakes are a breakfast staple, providing a little fruit inside a delicious pancake that your baby can eat with her fingers. The fruit usually softens easily during the cooking process, but if you are concerned about it being a choking hazard, you can process it a little to make a purple pancake batter.

 5 mins    10–15 mins   4 baby and 4 adult portions

## ingredients

1 **egg**
⅔ cup **buttermilk**,
  or ½ cup **natural yogurt**
  and ⅓ cup **whole milk**
¾ cup **self-rising flour**
1 tsp **baking powder**
1 tbsp **maple syrup**
  or 2 tsp **sugar**
1 tsp **vanilla extract**
5½oz (150g) **blueberries**
1 tbsp **vegetable oil**,
  for greasing

## method

**1** Preheat a griddle or non-stick frying pan over medium–high heat.

**2** Blend all the ingredients, except the blueberries, until smooth. Then stir in the blueberries.

**3** Brush the pan or griddle lightly with oil and spoon a few tablespoons of batter into the pan. For adult pancakes, use 2–3 tablespoons and 1 for baby pancakes. Cook the pancakes on one side, then carefully turn over to cook on the other side.

**4** When cooked on both sides, remove from the pan. Repeat the process with the remaining batter. Let cool a little before serving or storing.

✴ **Serve** *with cream cheese or a fruit purée (see pp59–62).*

✴ **Refrigerate** *in an airtight container for 24 hours or freeze.*

✴ **Variations:** *When apricots are in season, replace the blueberries with chopped fresh apricots.*

# Simple muesli

Rather than sugar-coated breakfast cereals, why not make this easy muesli for your baby? It provides essential iron and fiber and stores for a few days.

 5 mins      4 baby portions

## ingredients

½ cup **rolled oats**
2 tbsp **almond flour**
2 tbsp **unsweetened coconut**

½ cup dried **apricots**, chopped very finely.

## method

**1** Mix all the ingredients together and store in an airtight container.

**2** Serve with milk or natural yogurt.

✴ **Serve** *with milk and a few slices of banana.*

✴ **Store** *in an airtight container for up to 3–4 days.*

✴ **Variations:** *Apricots can be replaced with any dried fruit of your choice, including dried prunes, raisins, or dates. Chop them well as raisins can cause choking, especially if not softened.*

*Simple muesli*

# Savory muffins

Breakfast muffins don't need to be full of sugar, and this version sneaks in zucchini and cheese for a delicious starchy start to the day. They can also be served with soup or make a tasty snack. Conveniently, they freeze well.

 10 mins  12–20 mins  6 baby and 6 adult portions

## ingredients

¾ cup **all-purpose flour**
¾ cup **whole wheat flour**
3 tsp **baking powder**
3½oz (100g) **zucchini**, finely grated
2oz (60g) hard **cheese**, grated
1 tbsp finely chopped herbs such as **parsley, oregano or marjoram** (optional)
1 **egg**
½ cup **whole milk**
2 tbsp **vegetable oil**

## method

**1** Preheat the oven to 400°F (200°C). Grease a mini muffin and standard muffin pan, or line with paper liners.

**2** Sift the flours together with the baking powder into a mixing bowl, adding back any bran that remains in the sifter afterwards.

**3** Add the zucchini, cheese, and herbs, if using.

**4** Beat the egg in a bowl and stir in the milk and oil. Pour these over the dry ingredients to make a thick mixture.

**5** Spoon the mixture into the paper liners or pan. Bake for 12–15 minutes for the smaller muffins and 18–20 minutes for the larger ones.

✳ **Serve** *at breakfast with diluted fruit juice, eggs, or fresh fruit pieces.*
✳ **Refrigerate** *for up to 48 hours or freeze when cool.*

Nectarine slices

Savory muffins

# Carrot muffins

These light muffins provide essential calcium for a great start to the day. As with the savory muffins, these can be enjoyed at any time of the day and make a good transportable meal for days out.

 10 mins  12–15 mins  12 baby muffins

## ingredients

2 tbsp **vegetable oil**, plus extra for greasing
1 cup **self-rising flour**
1 **egg**
½ cup **whole milk**
2oz (60g) **carrots**, grated
1¾oz (50g) **hard cheese**, grated

## method

**1** Preheat the oven to 400°F (200°C). Grease a mini muffin pan or line with mini paper liners.

**2** Sift the flour into a bowl and add the egg, milk, and oil. Beat together with a blender or whisk to make a thick batter. Stir in the carrots and cheese.

**3** Spoon the mixture into the paper liners or pan and bake for 12–15 minutes, or until golden brown.

\*Serve *at breakfast with diluted fruit juice, eggs or fresh fruit pieces.*
\* Refrigerate *for up to 48 hours or freeze when cool.*

# Mango smoothie

Mangoes make a delicious smoothie that provides essential vitamin C. Serve to your baby in a lidded cup for her to sip.

 5 mins  4 baby portions

## ingredients

½ ripe **mango**, cut into cubes, or 5½oz (150g) mango cubes

½ cup unsweetened **pineapple** or **apple juice**

## method

**1** Blend the mango cubes and juice until smooth.

**2** Chill until required.

\*Serve *in a sippy cup as part of a main meal.*
\* Refrigerate *in an airtight container for up to 24 hours.*
\* Variations: *Add a ripe peach or nectarine, peeled and chopped in step 1.*

# Vanilla and banana smoothie

Breakfast in a cup for your baby, this easy to make, calcium-rich smoothie is bound to be popular.

 5 mins  1 baby portion

## ingredients

½ ripe **banana**, cut into chunks
⅓ cup **natural yogurt**

1–2 drops **vanilla extract**

## method

**1** Blend the banana, yogurt, and vanilla extract until smooth.

**2** Serve in a cup immediately.

\*Serve *as an accompaniment to a main meal.*
\* Not suitable for storage.
\* Variations: *Add 1–2 dried chopped apricots.*

# Baked egg with cheese and tomato

Oven-baked eggs make a nice change to hard-boiled ones, and your baby will enjoy the variety of flavors here.

 5 mins   🔥 10 mins   🥧 1 baby portion

## ingredients

**vegetable oil**, for greasing
½ **tomato**, halved, seeded, and finely chopped
1 **egg**
¼oz (10g) **Cheddar cheese**, grated

## method

**1** Preheat the oven to 350°F (180°C). Lightly grease a small flameproof dish, such as a ramekin.

**2** Place the tomato at the bottom of the dish and crack the egg over it.

**3** Sprinkle with the cheese and bake uncovered for around 10 minutes, or until the yolk has set.

＊ **Serve** *with pieces of buttered toast or bread.*
＊ *Not suitable for storage.*
＊ **Variations:** *Add a few chopped chives or a small quantity of shredded ham.*

# Corn and tomato fritters

These little fritters make a lovely weekend breakfast when you may have slightly more time to cook. It won't be just your baby enjoying them—you'll love them, too. By this stage, your baby will be able to cope with lumps so the corn shouldn't be a problem. If she is slow to chew, you can chop the corn a little in a processor.

 5 mins   🔥 5–10 mins   🥧 20 fritters   ❄️

Corn fritters

## ingredients

1 cup **self-rising flour**
1 **egg**
⅔ cup **whole milk**
1–2 tsp chopped **chives**
1 medium **tomato**, halved, seeded, and finely chopped
5½oz (150g) **corn kernels**, canned in water, or frozen and defrosted
1–2 tbsp **vegetable oil**

## method

**1** Make the batter by blending the flour, egg, and milk until smooth.

**2** Pour into a bowl and add the chives, tomato, and corn. Stir well to combine.

**3** Heat 1 tablespoon of the oil in a large non-stick frying pan. Spoon about 1 tablespoon of the batter into the hot oil and repeat until you have several fritters cooking.

**4** Cook for 2–4 minutes, or until golden brown on the bottom, then turn over and cook on the other side. Drain on paper towels and continue cooking until all the batter is used up.

＊ **Serve** *with a few halved cherry tomatoes.*
＊ **Wrap** *individually in plastic wrap and refrigerate for 24 hours or freeze when cooled.*

# Sardines on toast

Sardines are fantastically nutritious—high in zinc, iron, and B vitamins, and the soft bones provide calcium and vitamin D. Mash well to incorporate the bones.

 2 mins   3 mins   1 baby portion

## ingredients

1 slice **bread**
   of your choice
1 canned **sardine** in oil
   or tomato sauce
1 tsp **lemon juice** (optional)
**cucumber** slices

## method

**1** Preheat the broiler and toast the bread on both sides

**2** Mash the canned sardine well with the lemon juice, if using.

**3** Spread over the toast and broil for 2–3 minutes, or until bubbling and hot.

**4** Cool and cut into pieces. Serve with cucumber slices.

**\*** Note: *Mackerel or pilchards can be used instead of sardines. These oily fish retain their omega 3 during the canning process, unlike tuna.*

# Pineapple and cheese on toast

Pineapple and cheese is a delicious combination. Canned pineapple in juice is softer than the fresh fruit, so easier for babies to chew—and available whatever the season.

 2 mins   3 mins   1 baby portion

## ingredients

1 slice **bread** of your choice
1 tsp **butter** or **olive oil spread**
1 canned **pineapple ring** in juice,
   plus more to serve
½oz (15g) **Cheddar cheese**, grated

## method

**1** Preheat the broiler. Toast the bread and spread with the butter or olive oil spread.

**2** Cut the pineapple into small chunks and scatter over the toast. Then sprinkle with the cheese.

**3** Broil for 2–3 minutes, or until the cheese is bubbling and brown.

**4** Remove from the heat, cool slightly, and cut into pieces. Serve with more chunks of pineapple.

# Baked beans on toast

Did you know that baked beans combined with wheat toast provides a great mix of proteins for vegetarian babies? Not only that, but the beans provide iron, too. Choose salt- and sugar-reduced varieties of baked beans.

 2 mins   3 mins   1 baby portion

## ingredients

1 heaping tbsp **baked beans**
1 slice **bread** of your choice
1 tsp **butter** or **olive oil spread**

## method

**1** Heat the beans in a saucepan or microwave oven until they are piping hot. Pour into a little bowl and let cool to body temperature.

**2** Meanwhile, toast the bread and spread with the butter or spread.

**3** Cut the toast into pieces and serve with the beans.

# Ways with *sandwiches*

**Sandwiches make a simply prepared meal** that's both portable and easy for your baby to pick up. Your baby may manage one slice of bread cut in half and sandwiched together, or want more or less than this, depending on her appetite. Choose nutritious fillings that provide protein as well as vegetables. It doesn't matter if your baby has white, or whole wheat bread at this stage; in fact, it is a good idea to let her sample these different varieties now, then by one year she can branch out more and try breads with grains or seeds.

Ricotta, tomato, and basil

## Ricotta, tomato, and basil

### ingredients

1 heaping tbsp **ricotta cheese**
½ **tomato**, seeded and finely chopped
2 small **basil leaves**, shredded
1 slice **bread** of your choice
**carrot or cucumber**, cut into sticks, to serve

### method

**1** Mix the ricotta and tomato together, then add the basil.

**2** Spread these over the bread, and cut in half.

**3** Sandwich together, cut into small pieces or quarters, and serve the sandwiches with the carrot or cucumber batons.

Egg and cress

# Egg and sprouts

## ingredients

1 **egg**
1 tbsp reduced-fat **mayonnaise**
1 slice **bread** of your choice
1 tbsp **alfalfa sprouts**, finely chopped
**cherry tomatoes**, to serve

✱ *Extra egg mixture can be refrigerated in an airtight container overnight.*

## method

**1** Hard boil the egg by cooking in a saucepan of simmering water for up to 10 minutes. Remove and cool by dipping into cold water. Peel the egg and chop into a bowl.

**2** Stir in the mayonnaise and mix well to combine.

Spread over the bread, then sprinkle with the sprouts and cut in half.

**3** Sandwich together, cut into small pieces or quarters, and serve with the cherry tomatoes, halved.

# Tuna and avocado

## ingredients

½ small **avocado**
1 tsp **lemon** or **lime juice**
scant 1oz (25g) **canned tuna** in oil or water
1 slice **bread** of your choice
**cherry tomatoes**, to serve

## method

**1** Scoop the avocado into a small bowl, sprinkle with the lemon juice, and mash until soft.

**2** Stir in the tuna and mix well. Spread over the bread and cut in half.

**3** Sandwich together, cut into small pieces or quarters, and serve with the cherry tomatoes, halved.

Tuna and avocado

# Ways with *fillers*

**For babies approaching one year old,** self-feeding becomes less tricky, even if the mess is the same. Filled crêpes (p192), tortillas, and chapatis provide a new experience, and can be eaten as finger foods. These fillings can also be used in baked potatoes. Here's a variety of toppings that can be batch-cooked and frozen.

## Salmon, yogurt, and cucumber

A summery filling to use either cold or at room temperature, salmon provides essential omega 3 fatty acids.

🕒 5 mins    🔥 12–15 mins    🥧 6 baby portions

### ingredients

2oz (60g) cooked **salmon** (see p186)
2 heaping tbsp **full-fat natural yogurt**
½ tsp finely grated **lemon zest**
1in (3cm) piece **cucumber**, finely chopped

### method

**1** Check the cooked salmon for bones and flake into a small bowl. Stir in the yogurt, lemon zest, and cucumber.

**2** Chill until required or use immediately.

✳ *Not suitable for freezing. Must be eaten chilled within 24 hours.*

✳ **Variation:** *Replace the cucumber with ½ small avocado, cut into small cubes.*

## Spicy chicken and vegetables

Fill tortillas or crêpes and slice as finger food or serve the chicken in a bowl with pieces of crêpe or tortilla on the side.

🕒 5 mins    🔥 20–25 mins    🥧 6 baby portions    ❄

### ingredients

1 tbsp **olive** or **vegetable oil**
1 small **onion**, finely chopped
3½oz (100g) **boneless, skinless chicken breasts**, roughly chopped
¼ **red bell pepper**, sliced
3½oz (100g) **mushrooms**, sliced
1 x 7oz (200g) can chopped **tomatoes** in juice
pinch of **Cajun spices** (optional)

### method

**1** Heat the oil in a non-stick saucepan and cook the onion and chicken, stirring frequently, until the chicken is lightly colored on all sides.

**2** Add all the remaining ingredients and gently bring to a simmering point. Stir, cover, and continue cooking for 15–20 minutes until the vegetables are tender. Cool a little before using.

✳ **Refrigerate** *for 24 hours or freeze when cooled.*

✳ **Variations:** *Use 3½oz (100g) zucchini instead of the mushrooms. For the adult portion, add more Cajun spices.*

# Cheese and tomato

Simply cooked onion and tomato with a little cheese provides protein and vitamin C and makes a popular filling for tortillas. It can be varied in many ways.

 5 mins    15 mins    2–3 baby portions  

## ingredients

1 tbsp **olive** or **vegetable oil**
1 small **onion**, finely chopped
7oz (200g) fresh **tomatoes**, roughly chopped
pinch of **thyme**
½oz (15g) **Cheddar cheese**, grated (For each crêpe, baked potato, or tortilla)

## method

**1** Heat the oil in a small saucepan and gently cook the onion for about 5 minutes, or until lightly browned and slightly softened, stirring frequently.

**2** Add the chopped tomatoes and thyme and cook over medium heat for 10 minutes, stirring frequently, until the mixture is thickened and the tomatoes soft. Sprinkle with cheese, cool slightly, and serve, sprinkling cheese over the top.

✳ Refrigerate *for 24 hours or freeze when cooled.*

✳ **Variations:** *Use 7oz (200g) chopped canned tomatoes instead of the fresh tomatoes. You can also add ½ red or green bell pepper, finely chopped, or 1¾oz (50g) mushrooms, finely sliced.*

# Mexican beans

Beans are a good source of B vitamins and iron. Pinto beans are usually used in this dish, but other beans such as cannellini or kidney beans are good, too. Canned beans save time. Buy ones canned in water with no salt.

 5–10 mins    25–30 mins    2 adult and 2 baby portions  

## ingredients

2 tbsp **olive oil**
3½oz (100g) or 1 medium **onion**, finely sliced
2 **garlic cloves**, crushed
5¾oz (160g), or 1 **red** or **orange pepper**, diced
1 tsp **ground cumin**
1 x 14oz (400g) can **beans** in water, drained
2oz (60g) or 2 heaping tbsp **tomato paste**

For adult portions:
**Tabasco sauce**, to your taste
1–2 tbsp **jalapeño peppers**, chopped

## method

**1** Heat the oil in a non-stick saucepan and gently cook the onion and garlic for 5 minutes, or until softened.

**2** Stir in the pepper and cumin and continue cooking for another few minutes, stirring continuously. Add the beans, tomato paste, and 1¼ cups water, and bring to a boil.

**3** Stir, cover, and simmer for 15–20 minutes, or until the vegetables are tender. Take off the heat and cool a little.

**4** Remove about 3 rounded tablespoons per potion for your baby and process roughly to achieve a suitable texture. Let cool more while you add the Tabasco and jalapeños to your portion.

✳ Refrigerate *in an airtight container for up to 24 hours or freeze when cooled.*

# Ways with *pizzas*

**Make your own pizza toppings** for your baby's light meals using fresh ingredients. A halved English muffin makes a great base, but you could of course use a thick slice of bread or a halved bread roll.

🕐 5 mins　　🔥 6–8 mins　　◔ 1–2 baby portions

## Pesto, tomato, and mozzarella

### ingredients

½ **English muffin**
½ tsp **pesto**
3 **cherry tomatoes**, finely chopped
½ oz (15g) **mozzarella cheese**, diced

✳ *Serve with carrot, pepper or cucumber batons.*

✳ *Not suitable for storing.*

✳ **Tip:** *Pesto is salty, so use just a little. You can also replace the pesto with 1 teaspoon of tomato paste.*

### method

**1** Preheat the oven to 425°F (220°C). Spread the muffin with the pesto. Cover with the tomatoes and mozzarella cheese.

**2** Place on a baking sheet and bake for 5–7 minutes, or until the cheese is melted and just browning. Cool before cutting into pieces for your baby.

*Pesto, tomato, and mozzarella*

## Mushroom and onion

### ingredients

1 tsp **olive oil**
1 medium **mushroom**, finely chopped
2 **onion** slices, finely chopped

2 tsp **tomato paste**
pinch of dried **oregano**
½ **English muffin**
½ oz (15g) **Cheddar cheese**, grated

*Mushroom and onion*

### method

**1** Preheat the oven to 425°F (220°C).

**2** Place the oil, mushroom, and onion in a small bowl and cover with plastic wrap. Pierce with a knife before cooking on high for 40–50 seconds in a microwave oven to soften.

**3** Cool a little, and stir in the tomato purée and oregano. Spread over the muffin and sprinkle with the cheese.

**4** Place on a baking sheet and bake for 5–7 minutes, or until the cheese is melted and just browning. Cool before cutting into pieces for your baby.

✳ *Serve with carrot, pepper, or cucumber sticks.*

✳ *Not suitable for storing.*

✳ **Note:** *It is easier to cook the mushroom and onion mix in the microwave in a small bowl since the amount is little, but you can also soften on the stove in a small saucepan, if you prefer.*

# Tuna and tomato

## ingredients

2 tsp **tomato paste**
1 tsp **lemon juice**
¾ oz (20g) canned **tuna**, in oil or water
½ **English muffin**
½ oz (15g) **Cheddar cheese**, grated

\* *Serve with carrot, pepper, or cucumber sticks.*

\* *Not suitable for storing.*

\*Note: *Canned fish may be quite salty, so look out for tuna with the least salt.*

## method

**1** Preheat the oven to 425°F (220°C).

**2** Mash together the tomato paste, lemon juice, and tuna. Spread over the muffin and sprinkle with the cheese.

**3** Place on a baking sheet and bake for 5–7 minutes, or until the cheese is bubbling and golden brown. Cool before cutting into small pieces for your baby.

*Tuna and tomato*

# Ham and pineapple

## ingredients

½ **English muffin**
1 tsp **tomato paste**
¼ oz (10g) unsmoked **ham** slice
1 slice **canned pineapple** in juice, finely chopped, or 1 tbsp drained crushed **pineapple**
½ oz (15g) **Cheddar cheese**, grated

## method

**1** Preheat the oven to 425°F (220°C).

**2** Spread the muffin with the tomato paste and place the ham on top. Spread the pineapple over the top and sprinkle with the cheese.

**3** Place on a baking sheet and bake for 5–7 minutes, or until the cheese is bubbling and golden brown. Cool before cutting into small pieces for your baby.

\* *Serve with carrot, pepper, or cucumber sticks.*

\* *Not suitable for storing.*

\* Tip: *Ham can be very salty, so only use the quantity as suggested, and choose unsmoked ham or reduced-salt ham, if available.*

# Leek and potato soup

Homey and filling, leek and potato soup always hits the spot on a cold day, so get your baby used to eating this mildly flavored soup. Use reduced-salt stock or water, and then season your own portion at the table. Leeks supply the B vitamin folate as well as plant substances called polyphenols that protect the body from disease.

 10 mins   15–20 mins   2–3 baby and 3 adult portions  ❄

## ingredients

2 tbsp **vegetable oil**

1lb 2oz (500g) **leeks**, (approx. 3), trimmed, washed, and sliced

1lb 2oz (500g) **Russet potatoes**, peeled and diced

2½ cups well-diluted low-salt **vegetable** or **chicken stock**

1 tbsp **chives**, chopped

For each adult serving, add 1 heaping tsp **crème fraiche** or reduced-fat **sour cream**

## method

**1** Heat the oil in a large non-stick saucepan and cook the leeks and potatoes for 5 minutes, stirring continuously.

**2** Add the stock and bring to a boil. Cover and simmer for 10–15 minutes, or until the potatoes are tender. Add half the chives and purée until smooth.

**3** Remove your baby's portion and let cool to lukewarm.

**4** Season the adult portions and serve with the crème fraiche or sour cream, and the remaining chives.

✱ Serve *with Cheesy polenta "twigs" (see p108) or Cheese scones (see p104).*

✱ Refrigerate *in an airtight container for up to 48 hours, or freeze on day of cooking when cooled.*

# Butternut or pumpkin and tomato soup

Pumpkin or other squashes can be roasted easily, which brings out their natural sweetness. Butternut squash is a significantly better source of vitamin A than pumpkin.

 10 mins   45–50 mins   3 baby and 2 adult portions   ❄

## ingredients

10½oz (300g) prepared **butternut squash** or **pumpkin**, cut into large chunks

1 large **red onion**, peeled and quartered

9oz (250g) ripe **tomatoes**, halved

1 sprig of **rosemary**

2 tbsp **olive oil**

1¾ cups low-salt **vegetable stock**

pinch of **nutmeg**, to serve (optional)

2 tbsp **crème fraiche** to serve

## method

**1** Preheat the oven to 400°F (200°C).

**2** Place the squash or pumpkin, onion, tomatoes, and rosemary in a roasting pan and drizzle with the oil. Give the pan a good shake to mix the vegetables with the oil.

**3** Roast for 40–45 minutes, or until the vegetables are softened. Remove from the oven and cool a little.

**4** Purée half the vegetables with half the stock until smooth. Pour through a sieve over a clean saucepan, then repeat the process with the remaining vegetables and stock.

**5** Check the seasoning, adding a little nutmeg, if desired. Serve warm with a swirl of crème fraiche on top.

✱ Serve *with bread and butter pieces or homemade croutons (see below).*

✱ Refrigerate *for up to 48 hours or freeze on the day of cooking when cooled.*

✱ Make simple healthier croutons: *While the vegetables are roasting, cut 2 slices of any bread into ½in (1cm) cubes. Place on a baking sheet, spray with an oil mister, and bake for 10 minutes, turning once.*

# Carrot and cilantro soup

This classic soup is full of vitamin A, and your baby will enjoy dipping in bread crusts, pita bread or the Cheesy polenta "twigs" (see p108).

 10 mins  25–35 mins  6–8 baby and 2–3 adult portions

## ingredients

- 2 tbsp **olive oil**
- 1 medium **onion**, roughly chopped
- 1 **garlic clove**, crushed
- 1lb 10oz (750g) **carrots**, scrubbed and roughly grated
- 5 cups **water** or diluted low-salt **vegetable stock**
- 1 tsp **ground coriander**
- 2 tbsp **chopped cilantro**
- 1 tsp **half-and-half**, to serve (optional)

## method

**1** Heat the oil in a large saucepan and gently cook the onion and garlic for about 5 minutes.

**2** Add the carrots, stir, cover, and sweat for 5 more minutes, or until softened but not browned.

**3** Add the stock and ground coriander and bring to a boil. Stir, cover, and simmer for 15–20 minutes, or until the vegetables are soft.

**4** Remove from the heat and stir in the fresh cilantro. Blend the soup in batches until you have a smooth soup, being careful as the hot soup can scald.

**5** Cool until just warm, and serve a ladleful to your baby in a sippy cup with a handle to drink, or in a shallow bowl. Stir in the half-and-half to serve, if desired.

✳ Serve *with Cheesy polenta "twigs" (see p108), Cheese scones (see p104), or bread/toast pieces.*

✳ Refrigerate *for 48 hours or freeze on the day of cooking when cooled.*

✳ Note: *For adults, season with a little salt and black pepper.*

# Pea and mint soup

This nutritious pea soup has to be one of the easiest to make, and is superior to any bought soup! Rich in vitamin C and fiber, it is on the table in less than 20 minutes. An older baby can drink it from a cup; younger ones may enjoy dipping in bread fingers or cheese scones.

 3 mins  10–12 mins  2 baby and 3 adult portions

## ingredients

- 1 tbsp **vegetable oil**
- 1 medium **onion**, chopped
- 1lb 2oz (500g) **frozen peas**
- 2 cups low-salt **vegetable stock**
- 3–4 **mint leaves**
- **black pepper** and **freshly grated nutmeg**, to serve

## method

**1** Heat the oil in a non-stick saucepan and cook the onion gently until softened.

**2** Add the stock and peas and bring to a boil. Simmer for 5 minutes, or until the peas are just tender.

**3** Add the mint leaves and then remove the soup from the heat.

**4** Cool slightly before blending until smooth. Season with the black pepper and nutmeg, and serve.

✳ Serve *with a swirl of cream, if desired, Cheese scones (see p104), or bread and butter pieces.*

✳ Refrigerate *in an airtight container for up to 24 hours or freeze on the day of cooking when cooled.*

✳ Variations: *Add 2 handfuls of washed spinach in step 2 to provide additional iron and folate. For a creamier soup, replace half the stock with whole milk.*

# Homemade tomato salsa

Store-bought salsa usually has salt and chile, which aren't suitable for babies, so making your own with fresh ingredients gives you control over what to add, and homemade usually provides more vitamin C than store-bought. It will still taste quite strong because of the raw onion, which some babies don't enjoy, so you may want to try with a little less onion at first.

 10 mins    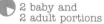 2 baby and 2 adult portions

### ingredients

9oz (250g) ripe **tomatoes**, washed, and halved
½ small **onion**, peeled and quartered, or 3 **scallions**, trimmed and quartered

½ small **red bell pepper**, roughly chopped (optional)
1 **garlic clove**, crushed
1 tsp **fresh cilantro**
1 tbsp **lemon juice**
**black pepper**

### method

**1** Blend all the ingredients and pulse until they are

roughly chopped. Be careful not to over-process them.

✳ **Serve** *with Turkey and red pepper patties (see p184), breadsticks, carrot sticks, or other vegetables.*

✳ **Refrigerate** *in an airtight container for up to 24 hours.*

Peach chutney

# Peach chutney

This is an easy fresh chutney that makes a great accompaniment to simply cooked foods, especially chicken or turkey burgers or fillets. When fresh peaches are in season use these, but otherwise you can use peaches canned in juice.

 5 mins   6 baby or 1 baby and 2 adult portions

 15–20 mins  ❄

### ingredients

2 tsp **vegetable oil**
½ small **onion**, finely chopped
1½oz (45g) **yellow** or **orange bell pepper**, seeded and diced
1 ripe **peach**, peeled, pitted, and finely

chopped, or 3½oz (100g) **canned peach** in juice
2 tbsp **water** or **juice**, if using canned peaches
1 tsp **wine vinegar**
1 tsp **brown sugar**

### method

**1** Heat the oil in a small non-stick pan and gently cook the onion and peppers for 5 minutes, or until softened but not browned.

**2** Add the peach, water or juice, vinegar, and sugar and

bring to a boil. Stir, reduce the heat, cover, and simmer for 10 minutes, or until the mixture has thickened.

**3** Cool to room temperature and serve.

✳ **Serve** *with Turkey and red pepper patties (see p184), Chicken burgers (see opposite), or Crispy salmon fingers (see p186).*

✳ **Refrigerate** *up to 24 hours or freeze on day of cooking when cool.*

✳ **Tip:** *To peel a peach, score a cross at the bottom and place in a heat-proof bowl. Cover with boiling water and leave for 20 seconds. Remove with a perforated spoon or tongs, and peel.*

Homemade tomato salsa

# Chicken mini-burgers with fruity sauce

A can of apricots in juice makes a sweet sauce to accompany these Thai-style mini-burgers. You can add chopped red chile or Tabasco to your portion.

 10–15 mins  15 mins  6 baby or 1 baby and 2 adult portions ❄

Chicken mini-burgers

## ingredients

9oz (250g) **ground chicken** (or process skinless **chicken breast** in a blender)
1 small **garlic clove**, crushed
1 tsp **lemongrass paste**
½ small **onion**, finely chopped
1 tbsp chopped **cilantro**

For the sauce
1 x 7oz (200g) can **apricot halves** in juice
½ small **onion**, finely chopped
1oz (30g) **golden raisins**
1 tsp **lime juice**
finely grated zest of ½ **lime**

## method

**1** For the sauce, drain the apricot juice and reserve it. Place 4¼oz (120g) of the apricots in a small pan with the onion, raisins, and ¼ cup of the reserved juice.

**2** Bring the sauce to a boil, stir, cover, and simmer for 10–15 minutes, stirring occasionally to break up the apricots. Preheat a broiler or griddle pan.

**3** Meanwhile, place all the burger ingredients in a bowl and mix to combine well. Divide into about 6 little patties, and flatten to ½–¾in (1–2cm) thickness.

**4** Broil or grill for 3–4 minutes on each side, or until the meat is cooked through and the juices run clear, not pink, when pierced with a knife.

**5** When the sauce is thickened, add the lime juice and zest; remove from the heat. For a lumpier sauce, mash; for a smoother sauce, blend briefly. Cool before serving.

✳ **Serve** *with mini-bread rolls and green or salad vegetables, either raw or steamed as appropriate.*
✳ *The sauce and burgers can be refrigerated for 24 hours or frozen. Freeze the burgers individually, separating each with plastic wrap or parchment paper.*

# Chicken and pasta with creamy sauce

This delicious dish is likely to become a favorite. Half-in-half with a fat content of around 10 per cent provides a creamy feel without adding too much saturated fat. The cornstarch stabilizes the sauce so it can be frozen.

 5 mins  12–15 mins  4–6 baby portions or 1 adult and 3 baby portions

## ingredients

2 tsp **olive oil**
2 **chicken mini-breast fillets,** or 1 small 3½oz (100g) skinless **chicken breast**, diced
1 small **garlic clove**, crushed
1½oz (45g) **button mushrooms**, sliced
1 tsp **cornstarch**
½ cup **half-and-half**
3 tbsp **whole milk**

1¾oz (50g) **frozen peas**, cooked
2 tsp **freshly chopped parsley**

Pasta
For each baby portion, use ½–¾oz (15–20g) dry weight **pasta**, such as pasta bows, penne, or children's pasta shapes

## method

**1** Boil the pasta in water according to package instructions, then drain.

**2** Meanwhile, heat the oil in a non-stick pan and cook the chicken over medium heat for 2–3 minutes, stirring frequently.

**3** Add the garlic and mushrooms; cook for 5 minutes, or until the chicken is no longer pink inside.

**4** Place the cornstarch in a small bowl and stir in the half-and-half and milk, then add to the pan with the peas and parsley.

**5** Bring to a simmering point, stirring continuously. When the sauce thickens, remove from the heat and cool slightly.

**6** Remove a portion for your baby and serve with the cooked pasta.

✳ **Refrigerate** *for up to 24 hours or freeze on the day of cooking in individual containers when cooled.*

# Turkey and red pepper patties

Turkey is a great source of vitamin B3, and peppers provide vitamins A and C, making this a nutritious finger food. It can be mashed for babies who prefer to be spoon fed.

 5 mins   14–17 mins   8 little patties

### ingredients

1 tbsp **vegetable oil**, plus extra for cooking
1 small **onion**, finely chopped
½ large **red bell pepper**, finely chopped
7oz (200g) **ground turkey**
1 tbsp chopped **parsley**
flour (optional)

### method

**1** Heat the oil in a non-stick pan and cook the onion and red bell pepper for 4–5 minutes, or until softened.

**2** Remove from the heat and cool a little before pulsing to combine with the turkey and parsley.

**3** On a clean cutting board, form 8 little patties; add flour if too sticky.

**4** Heat 1–2 tablespoons of vegetable oil in a non-stick frying pan, and gently cook the patties for 10–12 minutes, or until golden brown, turning over to cook on the other side. Remove from the heat, cool a little, and serve.

✳ **Serve** with Homemade tomato salsa (see p182) or Peach chutney (see p182).

✳ **Refrigerate** in an airtight container for up to 24 hours or freeze when cooled.

✳ **Variations:** Use chicken or ground pork instead of turkey. You can add garlic or herbs, such as tarragon, in step 2.

Turkey and red pepper patties

# Bulgur wheat with lamb and eggplant

Bulgur wheat is made by cracking the grains of either whole or husked wheat. Both provide protein and iron as well as dietary fiber. It's ideal for use in one-pot dishes where you can easily add it to stewed meat or vegetables.

 5 mins   20–25 mins   4–6 baby portions

### ingredients

7oz (200g) **lean ground lamb**
5½oz (150g) **eggplant**, finely diced
1 small **onion**, finely chopped
1 **garlic clove**, crushed
3½oz (100g) **bulgur wheat**
zest of half a **lemon**, finely grated
1 tbsp **tomato paste**
1 tbsp chopped **parsley**

### method

**1** Place the lamb and eggplant in a saucepan and cook over medium heat for 5 minutes, breaking up the lamb with a wooden spoon.

**2** When the lamb is lightly browned, stir in the onion and garlic and cook for another 5 minutes, stirring frequently.

**3** Add the wheat, lemon zest, tomato paste, and 1½ cups water and bring to a simmer. Stir, cover, and simmer for 10–15 minutes, or until the water has been absorbed and the wheat is tender.

**4** Remove from the heat, stir in the parsley, and let cool a little before serving.

✳ **Serve** with a green vegetable, such as spinach or broccoli.

✳ **Refrigerate** for up to 48 hours or freeze on the day of cooking when cooled.

✳ **Variations:** You can use ground beef instead of lamb. Add ½ teaspoon of cinnamon for a more Moroccan taste.

# Shepherd's pie

Shepherd's pie (made with lamb) or cottage pie (made with beef) makes an inexpensive nutritious meal. Rich in easily absorbed iron, this recipe is lovely for babies, toddlers, and adults. Make sure you use lean mince.

 15 mins      40–50 mins      2–3 baby and 3 adult portions     ❄

## ingredients

**vegetable oil**, for cooking
1 medium **onion**, finely chopped
1 small **leek**, finely chopped
1lb 2oz (500g) **ground extra lean beef**
3 medium **carrots**, peeled and diced
1¼ cups **water** or diluted **beef stock**
2 **bay leaves**

1 tbsp **cornstarch**

For the topping:
1¾lb (700g) **floury potatoes**, such as Russets, peeled and halved
3 tbsp **low-fat milk**
2 tsp **olive oil spread** or **butter**
**black pepper**

## method

**1** Preheat the oven to 400°F (200°C). Heat the oil in a large non-stick pan and add the onion, leek, and ground beef. Cook gently, stirring to break up the beef with a wooden spoon.

**2** Add the carrots. Cook until the beef browns and the onion softens. Add the water or stock and bay leaves, then simmer. Cover, reduce the heat, and cook for 15–20 minutes, stirring a little.

**3** Boil or steam the potatoes until tender. Drain and mash with the milk, olive oil spread or butter, and pepper. Mix the cornstarch with 2 tablespoons of cold water; add to the meat to thicken. Pour into a flameproof dish and remove the bay leaves.

**4** Spoon or pipe the potato; bake for 20–25 minutes, or until the mixture is piping hot and the potato starting to brown. Remove your baby's portion and cool a little before serving.

✳ **Serve** *with steamed broccoli, kale or cabbage.*
✳ **Cover** *and refrigerate for 24 hours or freeze on the day of cooking.*

# Beef meatballs in tomato sauce

Meatballs are a family favorite. Whether your baby likes to use her fingers, or to eat mashed meatballs from a spoon, you'll be providing her with an iron-rich meal.

 15 mins      25–30 mins      6–8 baby portions     ❄

## ingredients

For the sauce:
1 tbsp **vegetable oil**
1 small **onion**, peeled and finely chopped
1 **garlic clove**, crushed
9oz (250g) smooth **tomato sauce**
scant 1oz (25g) **sundried tomatoes** in oil, drained and roughly chopped
1 tsp finely chopped **thyme** or **oregano**

For the meatballs:
9oz (250g) **lean ground beef**
1 slice **whole wheat bread**
½ small **onion**, roughly chopped
few large **basil leaves**
**flour** (optional)
**vegetable oil**, for cooking

## method

**1** For the sauce, heat the oil in a non-stick saucepan and gently cook the onion and garlic for 4–5 minutes, or until softened.

**2** Add the tomato sauce, sundried tomatoes, and thyme or oregano, and bring to a simmering point. Stir, cover, and simmer for 15 minutes, stirring occasionally.

**3** For the meatballs, blend the beef, bread, onion, and basil until mixed. Form into 20 small balls, using flour if sticky.

**4** Heat 1–2 tablespoons of oil in a non-stick pan and cook the meatballs until browned, turning as they cook.

**5** Drain on paper towels. For each portion, serve 2–3 balls with 1 tablespoon of sauce.

✳ **Serve** *with rice, mashed potatoes, or pasta.*
✳ **Refrigerate** *for up to 24 hours or freeze in individual portions on day of cooking when cooled.*
✳ **Variations:** *Use any meat or ground poultry.*

Beef meatballs in tomato sauce

# Crispy salmon fingers

Crispy salmon fingers

Homemade fish fingers are quick to make, and using salmon provides your baby with important omega 3 fatty acids for brain and eye development. These are also ideal for babies who like to feed themselves as they can be held and dipped.

 5–10 mins  12–15 mins  6–8 fingers ✳

## ingredients

1 slice day old, half and half **bread** (50 per cent whole wheat), crusts removed

1 tsp finely chopped **parsley**
finely grated zest of ¹/₂ **lemon**
1 **egg**
3½oz (100g) skinless **salmon fillet**

## method

**1** Preheat the oven to 375°F (190°C). Line a baking sheet with a non-stick paper or parchment paper.

**2** Blend the bread into fine bread crumbs. Pulse as you add the parsley and lemon zest. Pour the bread crumb mix into a shallow bowl.

**3** Meanwhile, beat the egg in a shallow bowl.

**4** Check the fish for bones by running your finger over the surface; remove any you find.

**5** Cut into 6 or 8 small pieces. Carefully place one piece in the egg and coat it all over. Using tongs, transfer it to the bowl of bread crumbs and coat with crumbs. Place the coated piece on the baking sheet and repeat with all the fish.

**6** Bake for 6 minutes, then turn over to the other side and bake until crispy. Let cool before serving.

✳ **Serve** *with Avocado dip (see p106), Tomato salsa (see p182), and some halved cherry tomatoes.*

✳ *The fingers are a little fragile, but can be carefully frozen if separated by parchment paper.*

✳ **Variations:** *Any firm fish can be used for this, but oily fish contains more omega 3.*

# Salmon and dill risotto

Babies love rice, and whether they are spoon fed or like to get their hands sticky, this risotto provides great nutrition. Chopped frozen spinach is easy to stir in at the end of cooking, saving you time.

 5–10 mins  35–40 mins  3–4 baby or 2 baby and 2 adult portions  ✳

## ingredients

3½oz (100g) **salmon fillet**
juice of ½ **lemon**
1 tbsp **vegetable oil**
4in (10cm) piece white part of a **leek**, finely chopped
2½oz (75g) **risotto rice**
1¾ cups low-salt **vegetable** or **fish stock**
1 tsp **chopped dill**
2oz (60g) frozen chopped **spinach**, defrosted and drained
1oz (30g) **mascarpone** or **cream cheese**
**black pepper** and **salt**, to serve (optional)

## method

**1** Preheat the oven to 375°F (190°C).

**2** Check the fish for bones by running your finger over the surface and removing any you find. Place in an oven-proof dish and pour in the lemon juice. Steam, microwave, or bake for 12–15 minutes, or until the fish flakes easily. When cooked, remove the skin and keep warm.

**3** Heat the oil in a saucepan and cook the leek for 3–4 minutes, until soft but not brown.

**4** Add the risotto rice and stir in about ¹/₃ of the stock. Stir and continue cooking over medium heat, stirring in more liquid until all the fluid has been absorbed.

**5** After 30–35 minutes, or when the rice is tender and all the liquid absorbed, stir in the dill and spinach and heat through briefly. Remove from the heat and stir in the mascarpone. Flake the salmon into the risotto and stir to combine.

**6** Remove your baby's portion and serve. Season your portion with the pepper and salt, if desired.

✳ **Serve** *with halved cherry tomatoes, steamed cauliflower, or carrots.*

✳ **Freeze** *on the day of cooking when cooled.*

# Simple fish pie

Full of calcium, magnesium, and B vitamins, this potato-topped fish pie is a family favorite. It freezes well, so you can double the mixture and freeze half in a foil tray for days when you have less time to cook.

 20 mins    40–45 mins    2–3 baby and 3 adult portions

## ingredients

1lb 2oz (500g) skinless
   **white fish** fillets
2 cups **whole milk**
2 **bay leaves**
strip of **lemon zest**
**vegetable oil**, for greasing
2 tbsp **butter** or
   **monounsaturated spread**
2 tbsp **all-purpose flour**
3 tbsp **half-and-half**
3¼oz (100g) **frozen peas**, thawed
1 tbsp chopped **parsley**

### For the topping

1¾lb (700g) **Russet potatoes**,
   peeled and quartered
2 tbsp **whole milk**
2 tbsp of **butter** or
   **monounsaturated spread**

## method

**1** Preheat the oven to 350°F (180°C). Run your finger over the fish fillet to check for bones, removing any you find.

**2** Pour the milk into a shallow or frying pan and add the bay leaves, lemon zest, and fish. Cover and heat very gently to poach the fish.

**3** Meanwhile, steam or boil the potatoes until tender. Mash with the milk and spread or butter.

**4** When the fish flakes easily, carefully remove from the pan. Oil a shallow flameproof dish and spread the fish over the base. Remove the lemon zest and bay leaves, and strain the milk into a bowl for use in the sauce.

**5** To make the sauce, heat the butter or spread in a saucepan and stir in the flour. Cook for 30 seconds, then add the reserved milk, little by little, stirring constantly, until the sauce has thickened. Add the half-and-half, peas, and parsley and pour over the fish.

**6** Spoon or pipe the mashed potatoes over the fish. Bake for 25–30 minutes, or until golden brown. Remove your baby's portion and let cool a little before serving.

✳ **Serve** *with more peas, broccoli, and a few carrots.*

✳ **Cover** *with plastic wrap and refrigerate for 24 hours. Alternatively, freeze before baking, and when defrosted (best in the fridge overnight), bake as in step 6, allowing a little longer to ensure it is piping hot.*

# Bulgur wheat with currants and chickpeas

Bulgur wheat makes a moist dish with succulent currants and chickpeas. This is a meal in itself, although it can be served as an accompaniment to a casserole or broiled meat or poultry for older children and adults.

 5–10 mins    25 mins    2 baby and 2–3 adult portions

## ingredients

1 tbsp **vegetable oil**
1 medium **onion**,
   finely chopped
5½oz (150g) **butternut
   squash**, finely diced
scant 1oz (25g) **currants**
3½oz (100g) **bulgur wheat**
1 x 14oz (400g) can
   **chickpeas** in water, rinsed
   and drained
2 **bay leaves**
1 heaping tbsp
   chopped **parsley**

## method

**1** Heat the oil in a large saucepan and gently cook the onion for 5 minutes, or until just softening. Add the butternut squash and continue cooking over medium heat, stirring frequently for 5 minutes.

**2** Stir in the currants, wheat, chickpeas, 2 cups water, and bay leaves, and bring to a boil. Cover, reduce the heat, and simmer for 15 minutes. In the last few minutes of cooking, remove the bay leaves, and stir in the parsley.

**3** When the wheat is tender, remove from the heat and let stand for 5 minutes. Remove your baby's portion and let cool a little before serving. You can also mash, if required, to an appropriate consistency for your baby before serving.

✳ **Serve** *with steamed green beans, broccoli, or halved cherry tomatoes.*

✳ **Refrigerate** *for up to 24 hours.*

✳ **Variations:** *Use raisins instead of currants. Chickpeas can also be replaced with any type of cooked beans.*

# Cowboy beans with cornmeal topping

Cornmeal or fine polenta makes a lovely crust on top of spicy beans. Beans supply a host of different B vitamins, as well as some iron, and the vitamin C in the tomato sauce helps the iron to be absorbed.

 10 mins      35–40 mins      4 baby and 2 adult portions     ❄

## ingredients

1 tbsp **vegetable oil**, plus extra for greasing
1 small **onion**, finely chopped
2½oz (75g) **mushrooms**, halved and sliced
9oz (250g) cooked or canned **beans** of your choice, such as pinto, cannellini, or borlotti
14oz (400g) can chopped **tomatoes** in juice
2 tbsp **tomato paste**
1 tbsp chopped **thyme**

### For the topping:

2 large **eggs**
1¾oz (50g) fine **cornmeal** or **polenta**
½ cup **all-purpose flour**
1 tsp **baking powder**
**black pepper**
1¾oz (50g) **hard cheese**, such as Cheddar, grated (optional)

## method

**1** Preheat the oven to 375°F (190°C) and grease a medium-sized flameproof dish with the oil.

**2** For the beans, heat the oil in a non-stick pan and gently cook the onion for 5 minutes, or until softened, stirring frequently. Add the mushrooms and continue to cook for 3–4 minutes, or until the mushrooms soften.

**3** Add the beans, tomatoes, tomato paste, ½ cup water, and thyme. Bring to a boil, then carefully pour into the dish.

**4** For the topping, beat the eggs well with 3 tbsp water and stir in the dry ingredients. Add the grated cheese, if using.

**5** Pour the topping mix over the beans. Bake for 25–30 minutes, or until the topping is risen and firm. Remove your baby's portion and mash, if required. Let cool a little, and serve. Season your portion to taste.

✳ **Serve** *with a spoon of reduced-fat sour cream and steamed spinach.*

✳ **Refrigerate** *for 24 hours. The cooked bean mixture can be frozen when cooled separately or as a whole dish.*

✳ **Variations:** *For your portion, you can add chili sauce or smoky chipotle paste.*

# Creamy avocado pasta

This easy sauce can be made while the pasta cooks. Serve alongside the pasta for dipping, or chop or mash the sauce and pasta to a suitable texture for your baby.

 5 mins      12–15 mins      1 baby and 1 adult portion

## ingredients

3¼oz (90g) **penne pasta**
1 ripe **avocado**, halved and stone removed
2 tbsp **olive oil**
3–4 **basil leaves**, washed

grated **zest** of ½ **lemon**
2 tsp **lemon juice**
1¾oz (50g) **Parmesan cheese**, grated

## method

**1** Boil the pasta in water according to the package instructions.

**2** Meanwhile, scoop out the avocado flesh using a medium spoon and process

with all the other ingredients until smooth.

**3** When the pasta is cooked, reserve 1 tablespoon for your baby's portion. Season your portion to taste and enjoy!

✳ **Serve** *with a few halved cherry tomatoes.*

✳ *Not suitable for storage.*

# Fruity couscous with peanut sauce

Dried fruit, whether raisins, dried prunes, apricots, or currants, all provide iron. This can be served as a family side dish without the peanut sauce, but the peanuts provide protein, healthier fats, and iron, zinc, and copper.

 10 mins    10 mins    2 baby and 2 adult portions

## ingredients

5½oz (150g) **couscous**
1¾oz (50g) **currants**, or any dried fruit of your choice, finely chopped
5½oz (150g) **peas**, cooked

For the peanut sauce:
2 tbsp **coconut milk**
½ cup **crunchy peanut butter**, preferably salt- and sugar-free or reduced
1 **garlic clove**, crushed (optional)

## method

**1** Place the couscous and currants in a large bowl and pour in 1½ cups boiling water. Let stand until the water is all absorbed.

**2** Meanwhile, place all the ingredients for the peanut sauce together with ⅔ cup hot water in a small saucepan, and gently heat, stirring continuously, until the sauce is smooth and well combined.

**3** Stir the cooked peas into the couscous. Serve a portion of the couscous mixture topped with the peanut sauce.

✱ Serve *with a few halved cherry tomatoes. If your baby prefers, serve the peanut sauce separately with Flaked fish (p106) or Mini lamb and mint balls (p109).*

✱ Refrigerate *separately in airtight containers for 24 hours.*

✱ Variations: *Add corn instead of peas. For an adult sauce, add 1 tablespoon of soy sauce, 2 teaspoons of fish sauce, and 1 tablespoon of chopped cilantro when your baby has had her serving.*

# Vegetarian shepherd's pie

This potato-topped lentil and vegetable dish is a great source of plant-based iron. If you are bringing up your baby as a vegetarian, then don't forget to give her a well-diluted drink of unsweetened fruit juice with her main meals.

 15–20 mins    60 mins    8 baby or 2 baby and 2–3 adult portions

## ingredients

**vegetable oil**, for greasing
5½oz (150g) whole **lentils**
1 **bay leaf**
2 tbsp **olive oil**
1 medium **onion**, finely chopped
1 medium **eggplant**, cut into ½in (1cm) cubes
3½oz (100g) **mushrooms**, roughly chopped
1 tbsp freshly chopped, or 1 tsp dried, **marjoram**
1lb 10oz (750g) **Russet potatoes**
2 tbsp **whole milk**
1 tbsp **butter** or **olive oil spread**

## method

**1** Preheat the oven to 400°F (200°C). Grease a 2-quart (2-liter) flameproof dish.

**2** Rinse the lentils in a sieve, place with the bay leaf in a pan with cold water, and bring to a boil, simmering until softened. Timing varies with different lentils, so check the instructions. Drain, removing the bay leaf, and reserve some of the cooking liquid.

**3** Heat the olive oil in a large non-stick pan and cook the onion for 4–5 minutes, or until it starts to soften. Stir in the eggplant and mushrooms and cook over low heat for 10 minutes, stirring occasionally, and adding a little water, if necessary, to prevent sticking.

**4** Add the marjoram, the cooked and drained lentils, and ¾ cup of the reserved cooking liquid, with additional water, if required. Bring to a simmer, stir, and cook for 10 minutes, or until all the ingredients are fully softened.

**5** If the vegetables look large for your baby, blend half the mixture lightly and combine with the remaining mixture.

**6** Meanwhile, peel, quarter, and boil the potatoes until tender. Drain and mash with the milk and butter. Pour the lentil mixture into the dish and spread the mashed potato on top.

**7** Bake for 25 minutes, or until the top is lightly browned and the mixture piping hot. Cool a little before serving your baby.

✱ Serve *with steamed green beans, or broccoli florets or cauliflower.*

✱ Refrigerate *for up to 48 hours or freeze on the day of cooking when cooled.*

✱ Variations: *If you don't have time to cook lentils, buy cans of cooked unsalted lentils.*

*If you eat fish, use 1 teaspoon of Worcestershire sauce when you add the drained lentils.*

# Baked stuffed apple

In the US, Gala apples are traditionally used for this recipe, as their flesh becomes fluffy and meltingly soft. However, you can use any apple in season, just choose a sharp variety.

⏱ 5 mins    🔥 45 mins    🥧 2 baby and 1 adult portion

## ingredients

2 small **Gala apples**
2–3 tbsp **mincemeat pie filling**
1 tbsp **butter**

## method

**1** Preheat the oven to 325°F (170°C).

**2** Wash the apples and remove the core. Score around the circumference of each apple to prevent it from splitting while cooking.

**3** Place the apples in a small flameproof dish and fill with the mincemeat filling, pushing in as much as you can. Place a tablespoon of butter on top of each, and bake until the apples are really tender, about 5 minutes.

**4** Cool to just above room temperature. To serve, scoop out some of the soft flesh and filling, and place in a bowl. Mash if required.

✳ **Serve** *with vanilla ice cream or 1 spoon of natural yogurt.*

✳ **Refrigerate** *in an airtight container for 24 hours.*

✳ **Variations:** *Instead of mincemeat pie filling, use scant 1oz (25g) chopped dried fruit, such as raisins, prunes, or apricots, mixed with 2 teaspoons of dark brown sugar or maple syrup and a pinch of apple pie spice.*

# Baked spiced peach

Stone fruits such as peaches, nectarines, and plums make a deliciously simple dessert with minimum effort. Though baked, the peaches still provide plenty of vitamin C.

⏱ 5 mins    🔥 15–20 mins    🥧 2 baby portions

## ingredients

1 tsp unsalted **butter**, plus extra for greasing
1 **peach** or **nectarine**

1 tsp **brown sugar**
whole **nutmeg**, to grate

## method

**1** Preheat the oven to 400°F (200°C). Lightly grease a small flameproof dish.

**2** Peel the peach by pulling off the skin, or dip in boiling water for 20 seconds then remove. Halve the peach, remove the pit, and cut each half into 4–5 slices. Place in the dish.

**3** Sprinkle in the sugar and place the butter on top. Grate nutmeg lightly over the fruit and bake for 15–20 minutes, or until the fruit is tender.

**4** Cool and offer half the slices to your baby, storing the other half for another meal.

Baked spiced peach

✳ *Your baby may enjoy dipping these in natural yogurt.*

✳ **Refrigerate**, *covered in plastic wrap, for 24 hours.*

✳ **Variations:** *Plums or apricots can also be used instead of peaches, with the pits removed.*

# Stewed summer berries

This easy fruit compote is a rich source of vitamin C. Purple and red fruits are an excellent way to eat the protective plant substances polyphenols, which boost your baby's immune system.

 5 mins  5 mins  4–6 baby portions

## ingredients

7oz (200g) pack frozen mixed **summer fruit**, thawed, or an equivalent of fresh summer berries such as:
3½oz (100g) strawberries
1¾oz (50g) blueberries
1¾oz (50g) raspberries
3 tbsp unsweetened **apple** or **red grape juice**

## method

**1** If using fresh fruit, wipe with damp paper towels to remove any dust. Remove any stems from the strawberries and halve or quarter, if large.

**2** Place all the fruits in a small saucepan and add the apple juice.

**3** Bring very gradually to a simmering point and remove from the heat.

**4** Let cool, and serve at room temperature.

✱ **Serve** *with 1 spoon of Greek yogurt.*

✱ **Refrigerate** *in an airtight container for 2–3 days or freeze when cooled.*

---

# Exotic fruit salad

Fresh fruit provides an abundance of vitamin C and "phytonutrients": plant substances that boost health. Either cut up the fruit into larger pieces for your baby to hold, or chop up finely for spoon feeding. The fruit can be prepared and refrigerated for 24 hours, but add the banana just before serving.

 10 mins  3–4 baby portions

## ingredients

1 **kiwi fruit**, peeled and halved
2–3 slices of **mango**
1 small slice **cantaloupe**
2–3 tbsp unsweetened **pineapple juice**
few slices of ½ small **banana**

## method

**1** Cut the kiwi fruit either into slices or chop finely and place in a bowl.

**2** Cut the mango and melon into cubes, the size depending on your baby's needs, and add to the bowl.

**3** Pour in the juice, stir in the banana, and serve at once.

✱ **Serve** *with 1 spoon of yogurt or vanilla ice cream.*

✱ **Refrigerate** *in an airtight container for 24 hours.*

✱ **Variations:** *Add papaya or pineapple cubes.*

---

# Passion fruit and mango dessert

This is an idyllic combo. Although pricey, passion fruit makes a lovely addition to this creamy dessert. You can strain out the seeds, or leave them in for an older child.

 5 mins  2 baby portions

## ingredients

½ ripe **passion fruit**
2 tbsp **mango purée**
1 heaping tbsp **mascarpone**

## method

**1** Scrape the seeds from the passion fruit into a small sieve and press through the juice until you are left with seeds in the sieve. Discard the seeds.

**2** Pour the juice into a small bowl and mix with the purée.

**3** Beat the mascarpone with a wooden spoon until smooth, and carefully mix in the mango and passion fruit mix.

**4** Pour into 2 very small plastic bowls, cover, and chill.

✱ **Serve** *with fresh peeled mango pieces.*

✱ **Refrigerate** *in an airtight container for up to 24 hours.*

✱ **Variation:** *If including the passion fruit squeeze the seeds, omit steps 1 and 2, and once the mango and mascarpone are mixed, over the top. A little finely grated lime zest provides a nice zing for adults.*

# Mandarin gelatin

Sweetened only with the fruit and its own juice, mandarin gelatin is a nutritious alternative to shop-bought gelatin. Even with heat treatment, a can of mandarins provides a good source of vitamin C.

 5 mins     6 baby portions

*Mandarin gelatin*

## ingredients

10½oz (300g) can **mandarins** in fruit juice

¼oz (8g) or 1 heaping tsp unflavored **gelatin** unsweetened **orange juice**

## method

**1** Drain the mandarins from the can, reserving the fruit juice, and divide between 6 small dishes or one large one.

**2** Place 3 tablespoons of very hot, but not boiling, water in a small bowl and sprinkle over the gelatin. Let stand for 5 minutes, then stir until dissolved.

**3** Mix the reserved juice with the gelatin and enough orange juice to make 1¼cups. Pour into the dish(es) and refrigerate until the gelatin is set.

✳ **Refrigerate** *covered in plastic wrap, for up to 48 hours.*

✳ **Variations:** *Try a can of apricots in juice, adding any unsweetened juice of your choice. You can add a little grated fresh orange or lemon zest for a more citrus flavored tang.*

# Basic crêpe recipe

Using a very hot, well-used pan that doesn't allow batter to stick is the key to making good crêpes. The right pan means you don't need more than a dribble of oil for each crêpe.

 5 mins   10 mins   6 x 8in (20cm) crêpes   ❄

## ingredients

1 cup **all-purpose flour**
1 **egg**
1 cup **low-fat milk**
1 tbsp **vegetable oil**

✳ **Refrigerate** *for 24 hours or freeze on the day of cooking when cooled.*

## method

**1** Place the flour, egg, and milk in a blender or processor and combine to make a pouring batter.

**2** Meanwhile, heat a non-stick crêpe or frying pan until hot, and spoon in ½ tsp of oil. Bear in mind that hot oil expands so you won't need as much as you suspect.

**3** Swirl the oil around the pan and pour in a ladleful of batter, swirling this around the hot pan just to coat the bottom.

**4** Cook over medium–high heat until the batter has just dried, starts to peel away from the sides, and the bottom is lightly browned. Toss or turn the crêpe over and cook for another few seconds.

**5** Turn onto a plate and repeat steps 3 and 4 until all the batter is used up.

**6** The crêpes can be layered with waxed or parchment paper and frozen when cooled, or used fresh.

# Pear and raisin oat crumble

Crumbles are a favorite dessert, and the topping can be prepared and refrigerated for a few days, or frozen. The fruit base can be varied according to the season, and you could easily use plums, apples, or a combination of berries with these. Use unsweetened fruit juice to stew the fruit initially and only add sugar if necessary, as the topping contains sugar.

 10 mins  40–45 mins  2 baby and 3 adult portions

## ingredients

**vegetable oil**, for greasing
14oz–1lb (400–450g) or 3 **pears**, peeled, cored, and roughly chopped
1¾oz (50g) **raisins**
½ tsp **ground cinnamon**
3 tbsp unsweetened **apple juice**

For the crumble topping:
1 cup **all-purpose flour**
5 tbsp **butter** or **unsaturated margarine**
½ cup **rolled oats**
½ cup **brown sugar**

## method

**1** Preheat the oven to 375°F (190°C). Lightly grease a 1-quart (1-liter) flameproof dish.

**2** Place the pears, raisins, cinnamon, and apple juice in a saucepan and gently stew for 5 minutes, or until the pears begin to soften.

**3** Meanwhile, sift the flour into a bowl. Rub in the butter or margarine until the mixture resembles bread crumbs.

**4** Stir in the oats and sugar. Spoon the pear mixture and cooking juices into the dish and sprinkle with the crumble topping. Bake for 30–35 minutes, or until the crumble is crispy and a light golden color.

**5** Remove your baby's portion and ensure that it is not too much above room temperature before serving.

✴ **Serve** with 1 spoon of Greek yogurt, custard, or ice cream.
✴ **Refrigerate** for 48 hours or freeze when cooled.

# Apple sponge cake

Also known as Eve's dessert after Eve who took the apple from the tree of knowledge. And tempting it is, as it is a deliciously simple sponge cake topping with moist apples underneath.

 10 mins  30–35 mins  4 baby and 2 adult portions

## ingredients

**vegetable oil**, for greasing
10oz (300g) or 1 large **Gala apple**, or any other cooking apples
3 tbsp light **muscovado sugar**
grated **zest** of ½ **lemon**

For the sponge cake:
4 tbsp **butter** or unsaturated **margarine**, softened
¼ cup **superfine sugar**
1 large **egg**
½ cup **all-purpose flour**
2 tbsp **whole wheat flour**
1 tsp **baking powder**
few drops **vanilla extract**

## method

**1** Preheat the oven to 375°F (190°C). Lightly grease a 1-quart (1-liter) flameproof dish, preferably tall, not shallow.

**2** Peel and core the apple and slice finely. Mix with the muscovado sugar and lemon zest and sprinkle with 1 tablespoon of water. Spoon into the prepared dish and set aside while you make the sponge cake.

**3** Place all the sponge ingredients in a bowl and mix together well with an electric hand-held mixer.

**4** Spoon the prepared apple mixture over the top. Don't worry if it doesn't close up all the gaps as this will happen when it cooks. Bake for 30–35 minutes, or until the cake is set and the apple soft when pierced with a knife.

**5** Remove your baby's portion and ensure it is not too much above room temperature before serving.

✴ **Serve** with 1 spoon of Greek yogurt or vanilla ice cream.
✴ **Refrigerate** in an airtight container or freeze when cooled.
✴ **Variations:** Add a handful of raisins or other dried fruits, chopped, if large, to the apple mixture.

# Bread and butter pudding

A classic British pudding, bread and butter pudding is an economical way of using up day-old bread. It is also is a great way of providing a calcium-rich dessert that makes a change from Greek yogurt.

 5 mins    30–35 mins    2 baby and 1 adult portion

## ingredients

**vegetable oil**, for greasing
4 thin slices **white bread**
1 tbsp **unsalted butter**
1oz (30g) **raisins**
½ tsp **ground cinnamon**
1 large **egg**
⅔ cup **whole milk**
1 tbsp **superfine sugar**
**nutmeg**, to grate

## method

**1** Preheat the oven to 350°F (180°C). Lightly grease a shallow 2 cup flameproof dish.

**2** Remove the crusts from the bread, butter each slice on one side, and cut into triangles. Arrange a layer of bread on the bottom of the dish, with the buttered side facing up. Sprinkle in some raisins and cinnamon. Repeat the process, finishing with a layer of bread.

**3** Crack the egg into a bowl, then whisk in the milk and three quarters of the sugar. Pour over the prepared bread layers and grate over some nutmeg. Sprinkle over the remaining sugar and let stand for 30 minutes.

**4** Place the dish into the oven and bake for 30–35 minutes, or until the custard has set and the top is golden brown.

✳ **Serve** *with 1 spoon of natural Greek yogurt or a few slices of fresh fruit.*

✳ **Refrigerate** *in an airtight container for 24 hours.*

✳ **Variations:** *Any dried fruit can be used, chopped, if large. You can also use raisin or fruit bread, panettone, or brioche.*

# Apricot and almond upside-down cake

This upside-down cake is made with fruit and almond flour. Here, ripe apricots are used, or use canned apricots in juice, fresh plums, or peaches. Make a large family dessert or individual ones in ramekins.

 10 mins    15–18 mins    3–4 baby and 2 adult portions    ❄

## ingredients

**vegetable oil**, for greasing
2 large ripe **apricots**, halved
   and pitted
3 tbsp **superfine sugar**
2 tbsp **unsalted butter**

or **monounsaturated spread**
1 free-range **egg**
2 tbsp **all-purpose flour**
1 tsp **baking powder**
1 tbsp **almond flour**

## method

**1** Preheat the oven to 400°F (200°C). Lightly grease 4 small ramekins or one 5–6in (12–15cm) shallow flameproof dish.

**2** Cut the apricots into slices. Arrange at the bottom of the ramekin or dish.

**3** Beat together the sugar and butter in a small bowl until they are fluffy, and then beat in the egg.

**4** Sift the flour and baking powder and stir into the mixture along with the almond flour.

**5** Spoon the mixture over the apricots and bake for 15–18 minutes, or until the topping is lightly browned and bounces back when gently pressed. Cool, turn it upside down in a small dish, and serve.

*Apricot and almond upside-down cake*

✳ **Serve** *with natural yogurt or a scoop of ice cream.*

✳ **Refrigerate**, *covered with plastic wrap, or freeze on the day of cooking when cooled.*

✳ **Variations:** *Almond flour can be replaced with 1 tbsp all-purpose flour.*

# Blackberry apple cobbler

Fruit puddings do contain sugar and fat, but can be a good way to encourage fruit eating. This cobbler has a sloppy mixture that lets the fruit bubble up through the topping.

 10 mins   35–40 mins  2 baby and 3 adult portions

## ingredients

**vegetable oil**, for greasing
12oz (350g) or 1 large **eating apple**, peeled, cored, quartered, and sliced
5½oz (150g) **blackberries**, fresh or frozen
3 tbsp unsweetened **apple juice**
1 tbsp **sugar**, if desired

For the topping:
1¼ cups **all-purpose flour**
¾ cup **whole wheat flour**
2 tsp **baking powder**
4 tbsp **butter** or **unsaturated margarine**
¼ cup **superfine sugar**
grated zest of 1 **lemon**
½ cup **low-fat milk**
1 tbsp **brown sugar**

## method

**1** Preheat the oven to 350°F, (180°C). Lightly grease a 1-quart (1-liter) flameproof dish.

**2** Place the apple, blackberries, and apple juice in a saucepan and simmer for 5 minutes to begin to soften the fruit. Taste and add sugar only if necessary. Transfer to the flameproof dish.

**3** Meanwhile, sift together the flours and baking powder into a bowl, adding any remaining bran that remains in the sifter.

**4** Rub in the butter or margarine until it looks like bread crumbs. Add the superfine sugar, lemon zest, and mix in the milk to make a sticky mixture. Using 2 teaspoons, drop scoops of the mixture over the fruit and sprinkle with the brown sugar.

**5** Bake for 30–35 minutes, or until the scone mixture is cooked through and looks golden brown. Remove your baby's portion and ensure it is not too much above room temperature before serving.

✳ **Serve** *with 1 spoon of Greek yogurt, crème fraiche, or vanilla ice cream.*

✳ **Refrigerate** *for up to 48 hours or freeze on the day of cooking when cooled.*

✳ **Variations:** *Try with apple, berries of all types, or stone fruits.*

*Blackberry apple cobbler*

# Baked egg custard

This childhood favorite is high in protein and calcium, and easy to eat. Rather than cooked in a pie crust, these are baked in small ramekins that can be stored for 24 hours in the fridge.

 5 mins   15–20 mins   3 baby portions

## ingredients

**vegetable oil**, for greasing
1 **egg**
¼ tsp **vanilla extract**
2 tsp **sugar**
⅔ cup **whole milk**
**nutmeg**, to grate

## method

**1** Preheat the oven to 375°F (190°C). Grease 3 small ramekins or flameproof dishes.

**2** Beat the egg well in a bowl with the vanilla extract and sugar. Heat the milk until it is hot, but not boiling, and whisk into the egg mixture.

**3** Strain the egg custard into the ramekins and grate a little nutmeg over the top.

**4** Place the ramekins in a flameproof dish and fill the dish up to ½–¾in (1–2cm) with water. Carefully transfer to the oven and bake for around 15 minutes or until set, depending on the depth of the custard. Remove from the oven, cool, and serve or chill until required.

✳ **Serve** *with fresh fruits or Stewed summer berries (see p191).*

✳ **Refrigerate** *for up to 24 hours.*

# Toddler to *preschool*

Your independent toddler is rapidly developing her own tastes and preferences, which means it's as important as ever now to keep offering healthy foods that provide the range of nutrients she needs to grow and thrive. Continuing the good work of the first months of weaning will help cement healthy eating habits that will stay with your child into adulthood.

# Your child's *balanced* diet

**You may be breathing a sigh of relief that the early months of feeding are over** and your toddler is eating a range of foods, but this is not the time to let up on ensuring she has a nutritious, balanced diet. As your toddler joins in more with family meals, it can be easy to forget that, as with younger babies, toddlers have high nutritional needs. In fact, your toddler uses more calories than you do per pound of body weight. She needs calories not just for growth, but for her increased mobility too.

## Your energetic toddler

Once your child is up on her feet, she'll be burning off plenty of calories as she walks, runs, and starts to explore. This means her need for calories and other important nutrients such as protein, vitamins, and minerals increases. You need to ensure that the foods and drinks she has are nutrient-dense—which means that for every mouthful she receives a good dose of a range of important nutrients. There are various ways to achieve this:

- Offer two nutritious snacks, such as fruit slices, cheese cubes, or vegetable sticks with a dip, in addition to three meals a day. Think of snacks as healthy mini-meals, rather than a cup of applesauce and a cookie.

- Provide vegetables and nutrient-rich meat, poultry, and fish consistently at mealtimes, even if these are sometimes rejected.

- Continue to use full-fat cheese, yogurt, and milk in cooking until your child is two years, as these provide vitamin A, calcium, and calories.

- Introduce some whole-grain foods such as whole wheat bread and breakfast cereals, but avoid high-fiber cereals containing bran, which interferes with iron absorption.

- Continue to use vegetable or olive oil in cooking as these are high in healthier monounsaturated fats.

- If you offer cakes or cookies, stick to the recommended portion sizes (see pp200–203). These foods are high in calories and saturated fat and have few other useful nutrients, so ideally make healthier versions yourself.

- The toddler years are also a time when your child starts to assert independence. She may refuse foods she previously liked, as she learns there are less nutritious, but tasty foods available. This can lead to deficiencies in iron, zinc, and vitamins A, D, and C, so it's important not to be put off by this tricky phase and maintain the good eating habits you've already established. With some patience and by keeping mealtimes simple with a positive atmosphere and not giving in to demands, it's possible to get through!

### Fast food

Parents are often worried about whether or not toddlers should have fast food when eating away from home. For an occasional meal, fast food is not going to harm your child, but don't get into the habit of promising this as a treat or reward, as this undermines all the good work you've being doing at home, and make sure it is a rare, rather than regular, occurrence. The portion sizes provided are often far too big for young children, and a toddler may easily have a full day's salt allowance in one meal, or an excessive amount of saturated fat and calories.

You can, of course, make your own healthier versions of these types of meals at home.

# Getting enough vitamins and minerals

Surveys show that many toddlers in the US don't have sufficient iron and zinc, or vitamins A, C, and D in their diet. A lack of these vital nutrients at this developmental stage can have long-term effects on health and development.

- Inadequate iron in toddlers can cause iron-deficiency anemia (IDA). A toddler with IDA, which can develop as early as one year, may be pale, tired, and irritable, and, if untreated, may suffer delays in mental and motor development.

- Vitamin D is largely made by the action of sunlight on the skin and isn't found in many natural foods apart from oily fish. Inadequate vitamin D leads to the bone disease rickets, which can become apparent when toddlers begin to walk as their bones haven't developed properly.

- Zinc and vitamins A and C are all crucial for the development of the immune system, and other important functions.

You can ensure your toddler is getting essential minerals and vitamins by:

- giving vitamin drops that contain vitamins A, C, and D as recommended, unless your child is drinking a toddler formula fortified with these.

- including foods that are a good source of iron and zinc (see pp16–17).

- buying breakfast cereals fortified with iron.

- using fortified toddler foods and/or milk occasionally, especially if your toddler is a fussy eater.

You can help your toddler avoid IDA by:

- ensuring she doesn't drink large quantities of cow's milk, which is low in iron and can displace other foods from the diet. Between one and three years, a toddler needs only around 10oz (300ml) of milk as a drink per day.

- avoiding weaning late, and especially delaying the introduction of iron-rich foods.

- including good sources of iron such as red meat, fish or poultry in your child's diet.

- avoiding an over-reliance on beans, peas, and lentils or green vegetables to provide iron, as iron is less well absorbed from these types of food.

# *Toddler* portions

**As your toddler grows, her appetite increases** and she'll start to eat larger portions of foods. Parents often worry that their toddler will become overweight if they don't control what they eat. However, research shows that children need to learn to regulate their own appetite and will do this if they are allowed some control. Being over-restrictive and controlling won't allow your child to figure out when she is full, so offer a range of nutritious foods and let her determine how much of them to eat.

## Meeting your child's needs

It's helpful to have some guidance on appropriate portion sizes for different foods to help you get the balance right. The table opposite, based on information from The Infant and Toddler Forum, shows a range of suitable portion sizes for toddlers aged one to four years. Of course, all children have different nutritional needs, and the needs of an 18-month old will be different to those of a lively three year old.

### *Toddler drinks*

By now your toddler should be using a handled cup rather than a bottle for drinks. Whether with or without a lid will depend on her dexterity.

Cow's milk, which is not recommended under a year due to its low iron content, can be introduced now as a main drink provided your toddler eats well, with plenty of iron-rich foods. If she is a fussy eater, you may want to try one of the toddler formulas on the market that have added nutrients such as iron, omega 3, and vitamin D.

Continue to give water in preference to juice, especially between meals. Apart from contributing to tooth decay, too much juice, or milk, between meals can spoil her appetite. If you wish, unsweetened fruit juices diluted half and half with water at mealtimes will boost her vitamin C intake. Smoothies are best given at mealtimes too as these can fill her up and spoil her appetite; give just ½– ¾ cup.

### How much salt?

The table below shows some commonly eaten family foods and the amount of salt per serving they contain. Your toddler needs no more than 2g of salt a day up to the age of three. If she is eating family meals now, continue to avoid adding salt.

| FOODS | AMOUNT OF SALT (g) |
| --- | --- |
| Cow's milk – whole 3½fl oz (100ml) | 0.14 |
| 1 slice white/whole wheat bread ¾oz (23g) | 0.24 |
| Cheddar cheese 1oz (30g) piece | 0.5 |
| Natural full-fat yogurt 3½oz (100g) | 0.1 |
| Greek yogurt, flavored 3½oz (100g) | 0.05 |
| Baked beans, heaping tbsp | 0.35 |
| Tomato ketchup 1 tbsp | 0.4 |
| Small bag of potato chips 1oz (25g) | 0.6 |
| 1 bacon slice – unsmoked ¾oz (20g) | 0.4–0.5 |
| Ham – small slice ¼oz (10g) | 0.2 |
| Bag of baked chips scant 1oz (25g) | 0.3 |

| TYPE OF FOOD | EXAMPLE | RANGE OF PORTION SIZES |
|---|---|---|
| BREADS AND SIMILAR FOODS | Bread roll | ¼–¾ roll |
| | Slices of bread/toast | ½–1 slice |
| | Naan bread | ⅛–¼ naan |
| | Chapati | ½–1 chapati |
| | Scone – fruit or plain | ½–1 small |
| | Teacake/fruited bun | ½–1 teacake/bun |
| | Breadsticks | 1–3 large breadsticks |
| | Rice cakes | 1–3 medium rice cakes |
| BREAKFAST CEREALS | Flaked cereals | 3–6 tablespoons |
| | Muesli | 2–4 tablespoons |
| | Teething biscuits | ½–1½ biscuits |
| | Oatmeal 'made up' | 5–8 tablespoons |
| GRAINS AND PASTA (COOKED) | Couscous | 2–4 tablespoons |
| | Rice | 2–5 tablespoons |
| | Pasta, plain or egg | 2–5 tablespoons |
| | Noodles | ½–1 cup |
| POTATOES | Baked potato | ¼–½ medium |
| | Boiled potato | ½–1½ egg size potato |
| | Mashed potato | 1–4 tablespoons |
| | Potato fingers | 4–8 thick-cut fingers |
| | Roast potato | ½–1 potato |
| VEGETABLES | Broccoli/cauliflower | 1–4 small florets |
| | Cabbage | 1–3 tablespoons |
| | Spinach, kale, or spring greens | 1–2 tablespoons |
| | Carrots – cooked | 1–3 tablespoons |
| | Carrot sticks | 2–6 sticks |
| | Celery, cucumber, bell pepper, or other salad vegetables | 4–10 sticks or slices |
| | Tomatoes | ¼–1 small tomato |
| | Cherry tomatoes | 1–4 tomatoes |
| FRUITS | Apple | ¼–½ medium apple |
| | Avocado | ½–2 tablespoons |
| | Banana | ½–1 medium banana |
| | Clementine or similar | ½–1 fruit |
| | Dried apricot/prune | 1–4 whole fruit |
| | Grapes or berries | 3–10 small berries |
| | Kiwi, plum, or apricots | ½–1 fruit |
| | Orange | ¼–½ orange |
| | Peach or nectarine | ½–1 whole fruit |

| TYPE OF FOOD | EXAMPLE | RANGE OF PORTION SIZES |
|---|---|---|
| FRUITS (continued) | Pear | ¼–¾ whole fruit |
| | Raisins/golden raisins | ½–1 tablespoon |
| | Fruit salad | 1 small bowl |
| | Stewed fruit | 2–4 tablespoons |
| MILK AND MILKY DESSERTS | Full-fat cow's milk | 3–4oz (100–120ml) |
| | Custard | 5–7 tablespoons |
| | Rice pudding/semolina | 4–6 tablespoons |
| YOGURT | Greek yogurt, natural yogurt, or calcium-enriched soy dessert | 4½oz (125g) |
| CHEESE | Grated cheese in sandwich or pizza | 2–4 tablespoons |
| | Cottage or ricotta cheese | ½–1 tablespoon |
| | Processed cheese | 1 slice/triangle |
| MEAT AND POULTRY | Beef or lamb, sliced | ½–1 slice |
| | Pork, chicken, or turkey, sliced | 1–2 small slices |
| | Stewed ground meat | 2–5 tablespoons |
| | Lamb's liver | ½–1 slice |
| | Liver pâté | 1–2 tablespoons |
| | Bacon | ¼–1 slice |
| | Burger | ½–1 small burger |
| | Chicken nuggets | 2–4 nuggets |
| | Sausages | ½–1 medium sausage |
| FISH | Fresh or frozen white or oily | ¼ to one small fillet 1–3 tablespoons |
| | Canned fish in a sandwich/salad | ½–1½ tablespoons |
| | Fish fingers | 1–2 fingers |
| | Shellfish—shrimp | ½– 2 tablespoons |
| EGGS | Poached, fried, or boiled | ½ to 1 egg |
| | Scrambled egg | 2–4 tablespoons |
| | Omelet or frittata | Equivalent to 1 egg |
| NUTS | Ground, chopped, or crushed | 1–2 tablespoons |
| | Nut butters | ½–1 tablespoon |
| LEGUMES (BEANS, LENTILS, AND PEAS) | Baked beans in sauce | 2–5 tablespoons |
| | Chickpeas/hummus | 1–2 tablespoons |
| | Falafel | 1–3 mini falafel (1oz/25g each) |
| | Dhal/cooked lentils | 2–5 tablespoons |
| | Cooked or canned beans | 1–2 tablespoons |
| CASSEROLES, STEWS, CURRIES, AND STIR FRIES | Meat/fish/chicken/ beans with vegetable sauce and potatoes | 3–6 tablespoons |

| TYPE OF FOOD | EXAMPLE | RANGE OF PORTION SIZES |
|---|---|---|
| CASSEROLES, STEWS, CURRIES, AND STIR FRIES | Meat/fish/chicken/beans with vegetable sauce. No potatoes | 2–5 tablespoons |
| PASTA DISHES | Lasagna or macaroni and cheese | 2–5 tablespoons |
| | Spaghetti bolognaise | 3–5 tablespoons |
| PIZZA | Any topping | 1–2 small slices; 2½oz (70g) |
| POTATO TOPPED PIES | Shepherd's pie | 2–5 tablespoons |
| | Fish pie | 2–5 tablespoons |
| PASTRIES | Quiche or egg flan | ½–1½ small slices: 1–3oz (30-90g) |
| | Samosa | 1–2 small samosas |
| | Sausage roll | 1–3 mini rolls |
| SOUPS | Vegetable soup | 1 small bowl ½ cup |
| | Soup with meat, fish or pulses | 1 small bowl ½ cup |
| DESSERT * | Gelatin | 2–4 tablespoons |
| | Ice cream | 2–3 heaping tablespoons |
| | Fruit sorbet | 2–4 tablespoons |
| | Crêpe | ½–1 small crêpe |
| | Trifle or similar | 2–4 tablespoons |
| | Cake style dessert, for example apple sponge cake, or fruit crumble | 2–4 tablespoons |
| CAKES AND SWEETS * | Cupcake | ½–1 of a 1oz (25g) cake |
| | Muffin | ⅛–¼ of a 1½oz (125g) muffin |
| | Fruit pie | 1 small slice |
| | Danish pastry/pain au chocolat | ¼–½ medium pastry |
| | Plain croissant | ½–1 croissant; |
| COOKIES AND BREAKFAST SWEETS * | Granola bar | ½–1 bar; 1oz (20g) |
| | Graham crackers | ½–1 cracker |
| | Shortbread cookies | 1–2 cookies |
| | Chocolate sandwich cookie | ½–1 cookie |
| CONFECTIONERY ** | Chocolate bar/cookie | 2–4 small square or 1 funsize |
| | Chocolate buttons | 6–8 small buttons |
| | Popcorn, sweet | 1 small cup |
| CHIPS ** | Chips or savory puffed shapes | 4–6 chips or shapes |
| | Tortilla chips | 4–6 chips |
| | French fries—thin from fast food | 6–10 fries |
| | Poppadums | ½–1 poppadum |

\* These foods are high in energy and low in nutrients so observe the serving sizes. Include cakes or cookies with fruit as a dessert. They can be eaten twice a day in these portion sizes.

\*\* Confectionery and savory snacks can be offered once or twice a week as part of a meal. Don't use them as rewards, treats, or for comfort.

# Fussy eaters

**Some time in their toddler years,** most children decide that foods they previously ate are no longer acceptable. They may also become unwilling to try new foods, a phase called "neophobia," or fear of the new. This is a perfectly normal part of development as children learn to assert their independence, but can be very frustrating for parents who have spent time cooking nutritious meals, only to have them rejected or even thrown on the floor! Fussy eating is often a passing phase, and if your child is growing normally, it is not worth getting overly stressed. That may be easier said than done, but if you show your toddler it is upsetting you, it may be counterproductive, so try to stay calm, and keep offering nutritious meals and snacks.

## What can you do?

There are plenty of tactics to try to combat fussy eating:

- Keep an eye on what your child is eating or drinking between meals. Sometimes toddlers drink too much milk between meals, which can spoil their appetite.

- Sit and eat the same meal as your toddler; it is always nicer to eat alongside someone. Don't forget that you are your child's role model, so watching you eat can positively influence her.

- Be positive and calm. Offer your child food, and if it is not eaten, just take it away without comment after 15 minutes or so.

- Don't resort to bribes or persuasion. This can reinforce negative messages for your child. "You can have dessert if you eat your meat and vegetables" makes sweet dessert seem much more attractive than nasty vegetables.

- Don't insist that your child eat. If she is hungry she will eat, so make sure you offer nutritious food at mealtimes and for snacks, and don't let her fill up on milk and other foods between meals.

- Don't worry if your child goes through a phase of wanting only familiar foods. Continue to offer a range of foods, including the familiar food, and simply take food away if it's left uneaten. Toddlers like familiarity, especially if there has been a change, such as a new sibling, a move, or a new nursery, and a familiar food may help to settle them. This phase will normally pass quite quickly.

- If you're really struggling with mealtimes, ask your partner, relative, or a friend to take over occasionally. It may help to diffuse the tension you are feeling.

- Don't become over stressed about small issues. Some children don't like foods to touch one another or be covered with sauce or gravy—they like to see what they are eating. If this isn't too difficult just go with the flow, but if it becomes an issue, do talk to a health professional about it.

> *If your child rejects foods, try not to get too disheartened; continue to offer nutritious foods daily.*

# Small is beautiful

If your toddler seems overwhelmed when presented with a big bowl full of food, keep on offering small selections of food, as shown below, which she may find easier to cope with. If she manages to eat the smaller portion, you can always offer her more. Pages 200–203 list the average portion sizes for young children.

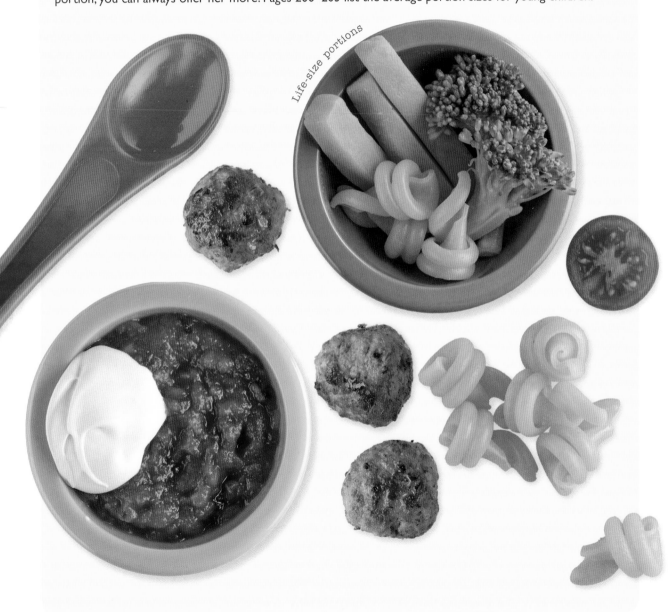

Life-size portions

# *Family* meal planner

By now, your little one will be enjoying **family meals** with the rest of the family much of the time. The two sample planners here offer some ideas for nutritious meals to suit the whole family. Snacks are also included as these are an important part of your toddler's diet now. Her little tummy can cope with only small amounts at a time, so to meet her energy needs now that she consumes less milk, she needs to eat smaller, more frequent meals.

## Monday

**Breakfast**
Simple muesli p169 with milk and slices of banana

**Mid-morning snack**
Half a buttered currant bun

**Lunch**
Half a small baked potato with grilled chicken thigh
Healthier coleslaw p211
Fruit yogurt

**Mid-afternoon snack**
2–3 dried apricots

**Dinner**
Tuna noodle casserole p218 with green beans or broccoli
Stewed apple and cranberries p129 and custard

## Tuesday

**Breakfast**
Teething biscuit p70 with raisins and slices of banana

**Mid-morning snack**
Apple slices

**Lunch**
Pea and mint soup p181 with cheese scone p104
Clementine or grapes

**Mid-afternoon snack**
Breadsticks and cottage cheese dip p107

**Dinner**
Mild chili con carne p217 with rice
Carrot and raisin salad p213
Baked spiced peaches p190 and yogurt

## Wednesday

**Breakfast**
Bircher muesli p98

**Mid-morning snack**
Mixed berry smoothie p168

**Lunch**
Scrambled egg p99 on toast with halved cherry tomatoes
Greek yogurt

**Mid-afternoon snack**
Halved grapes

**Dinner**
Chicken korma p213 with rice and cauliflower or peas
Passion fruit and mango dessert p191

## Thursday

**Breakfast**
Hard-boiled egg with buttered toast p69
Clementine or peach slices

**Mid-morning snack**
Half a buttered scone

**Lunch**
Whole grain salad p211 with a spoon of ricotta cheese
Appley plums p129

**Mid-afternoon snack**
Banana slices

**Dinner**
Salmon in filo pastry p218 with new potatoes
Sugar snap and apple salad p210
Chocolate rice pudding p135

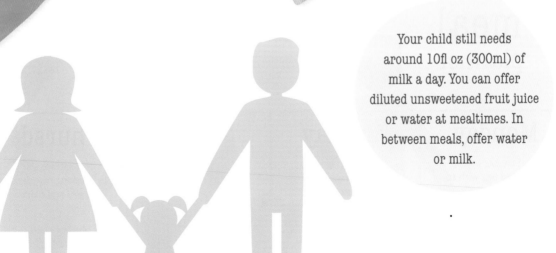

Your child still needs around 10fl oz (300ml) of milk a day. You can offer diluted unsweetened fruit juice or water at mealtimes. In between meals, offer water or milk.

# Friday

Breakfast
Raspberry oatmeal p99 with berries

Mid-morning snack
Pear or peach slices

Lunch
Tuna and avocado sandwich p175 with carrot sticks
Banana custard p133

Mid-afternoon snack
Rice cake with peanut butter

Dinner
Moussaka p215 with potatoes, broccoli, or corn
Fruit fool p133

# Saturday

Breakfast
Scrambled egg p99 on toast with clementine or strawberry slices

Mid-morning snack
Cinnamon spice pancakes p99

Lunch
Sweet potato, barley, and leek soup p102 with fingers of bread
Stewed summer berries p191 with yogurt

Mid-afternoon snack
Cubes of cheese

Dinner
Simple fish pie p187 with peas or corn
Mandarin gelatin p192

# Sunday

Breakfast
Spicy banana toast p100
Dried apricots or prunes, halved

Mid-morning snack
Carrot muffin p171

Lunch
Macaroni and cheese p125 with halved cherry tomatoes
Mango ice pop p132

Mid-afternoon snack
Red pepper sticks with homemade hummus p111

Dinner
Pork with plums p214 with roast potatoes, broccoli, and carrots
Chocolate rice pudding p135

# Beet and yogurt salad

Buy cooked beets from the supermarket, or just boil peeled beets and cool before mixing with an herby tangy yogurt dressing. Beet is a great source of the B vitamin folate, as well as being high in potassium.

 5 mins       2 toddler and 2–3 adult portions

Beet and yogurt salad

## ingredients

9oz (250g) cooked peeled **beets** (not pickled)
3 tbsp **Greek yogurt**

1 tbsp chopped **dill**
1 tbsp chopped **thyme**
juice of ½ **lemon**
grated zest of ½ **lemon**

## method

**1** Slice the beets, and then cut each slice into matchstick-sized pieces.

**2** Mix the yogurt with the herbs, lemon juice, and the zest, and stir in the beets. Serve, or chill until ready to serve.

\* **Serve** *with grilled chicken or fish.*

\* **Refrigerate** *for up to 24 hours.*

\* **Variations:** *Add ½ small red onion, finely chopped, and 1 small apple, cored and finely chopped.*

# Sugar snap and apple salad

Sugar snaps provide vitamin C in abundance, and the pods are rich in phytonutrients, which protect the body from disease. You can also use snow peas for this salad, which has the same nutritional benefits.

 5–10 mins    3–4 mins    1–2 toddler and 3 adult portions

## ingredients

7oz (200g) **sugar snaps** or **snow peas**
1 large red **apple**, washed
1¾oz (50g) **baby spinach** or other salad leaves, washed
1 tbsp toasted **sunflower seeds** (optional)

For the dressing:
1 tbsp **lemon juice**
1 tbsp **olive oil**
1 tsp **honey**

## method

**1** Trim the sugar snaps or snow peas and steam for 3–4 minutes. Dip into cold water to cool, then drain.

**2** Make the dressing by whisking all the ingredients together in a bowl.

**3** Quarter the apple, remove the core, and cut into small cubes. Stir into the dressing immediately. Cut the sugar snaps into slices around ½in (1cm) in width and mix into the dressing.

**4** Arrange the salad leaves on a serving plate, and spoon the mixture over it. Sprinkle with the sunflower seeds, if using, and serve at once.

\* **Serve** *with a summer barbeque or family dish, such as moussaka (see p215) or lasagna (see p217).*

\* *Not suitable for storing. Serve within a couple of hours of making.*

# Greek-style salads

Colorful and crunchy, Greek salad suggests the essence of summer—Mediterranean warmth, and the sunny flavors of ripe tomatoes and extra virgin olive oil. Keep the salad simple, using just olive oil to dress, and as the feta is salty, don't overdo this. In keeping with the theme, this salad is accompanied by a Greek-style leaf salad.

 5–8 mins       1 toddler and 2 adult portions

## ingredients

⅓ **cucumber**, halved lengthwise and thickly sliced

2 large ripe **tomatoes**, cut into chunks

1 small **red onion**, thinly sliced

3½oz (100g) **feta cheese**, cubed

scant 1oz (25g) pitted **black olives**

1 tbsp **olive oil**

For the leaf salad:
8 round **(butterhead) lettuce leaves**
2–3 sprigs of **dill**

For the dressing:
1 tbsp olive oil
2 tsp **red wine vinegar**
pinch of **sugar**
**black pepper**, to taste

## method

**1** Make the Greek salad by arranging the cucumber, tomatoes, onion, and feta in a salad bowl. Sprinkle in the olives and drizzle with the oil. Cover and set aside while making the other salad.

**2** Wash, dry, and gently tear the butterhead leaves and arrange in a salad bowl. Chop the dill and sprinkle this over the lettuce.

**3** Make the dressing by combining all the ingredients and pouring over the salad. Serve both salads together.

\* **Serve** *with whole wheat pita bread.*

\* *Not suitable for storing.*

# Healthier coleslaw

Store-bought coleslaw is usually made with fatty mayonnaise, making perfectly healthy vegetables go from low fat to high fat. This version uses very low-fat mayonnaise mixed with natural yogurt, which radically cuts the fat content while providing the same taste experience.

 10 mins       2 toddler and 2–3 adult portions

## ingredients

2 heaping tbsp low-fat (3 percent fat or less) **mayonnaise**

2 heaping tbsp **natural yogurt**

7oz (200g) piece **white cabbage**

2 medium **carrots**, peeled

2 sticks **celery**, trimmed and

washed

1¾oz (50g) **raisins**, or dried sweetened **cranberries**

1 tbsp **lemon** or **lime juice**

**black pepper**, to taste (optional)

## method

**1** Mix the mayonnaise and yogurt in a large bowl. Shred the cabbage very finely and add to the bowl.

**2** Coarsely grate the carrots, finely chop the celery, and mix into the bowl.

**3** Stir in the raisins or cranberries and lemon juice, and season with the black pepper, if desired. Cover and chill until required.

\* **Serve** *with baked potatoes, broiled meat, or poultry.*

\* **Refrigerate** *in an airtight container for up to 24 hours.*

*Healthier coleslaw*

# Whole grain salad

This colorful vitamin-C rich salad is a great accompaniment to grilled chicken or fish. This version uses quinoa, but it can be made with brown rice, barley, bulgur wheat or whole grain couscous. Just cook the grain according to the instructions and mix with the other ingredients.

 10 mins     10–12 mins     2 toddler and 2–3 adult portions

## ingredients

4½oz (120g) **quinoa**
7oz (200g) ripe **cherry tomatoes**, quartered
1 medium **yellow** or **orange bell pepper**, finely diced

1 heaping tbsp **basil leaves**, finely chopped or torn
2 tbsp **extra virgin olive oil**
**black pepper**, to taste

## method

**1** Cook the quinoa in unsalted boiling water according to the package instructions; drain in a sieve and rinse with cold water to cool.

**2** Place the quinoa in a serving bowl and stir in all the remaining ingredients. Serve at once, or cover and chill for use later the same day.

✳ **Serve** *with grilled chicken thighs and Healthier coleslaw (see p211) for a delicious summer meal.*

✳ **Refrigerate** *and use within 24 hours.*

✳ **Variations:** *Try peppers of different colors. Replace the oil with ¼ cup drained sundried tomatoes in oil and 1 tablespoon of the accompanying oil.*

*Whole grain salad*

# Pasta, tuna, and corn salad

A family standby, readily eaten by all, this salad has two alternative dressings, one the more traditional creamy tomato one, the other a fresher lemony one.

 10 mins     10–12 mins     1–2 toddler and 3 adult portions

## ingredients

7oz (200g) **pasta bows** or other shapes
5½oz (150g) **corn**, canned in water, or frozen
1 x 8oz (225g) can **tuna** in water, drained and flaked
4 **scallions**, trimmed and finely sliced

For dressing 1:
2 tbsp **reduced-fat mayonnaise**
2 tbsp **Greek yogurt**

1 tbsp **tomato paste**
1 tsp **lemon juice**
**black pepper**, to taste

For dressing 2:
1 tbsp **lime** or **lemon juice**
1 tbsp **olive oil**
½ tsp **superfine sugar**
**black pepper**, to taste

To finish:
1 tbsp chopped **parsley**
2 tbsp **pine nuts**, toasted (optional)

## method

**1** Cook the pasta in boiling water until just tender, then drain. Rinse in cold water and drain again thoroughly.

**2** If using frozen corn, boil for 2–3 minutes, drain, and cool. Mix the pasta, corn, and tuna in a large bowl, and add the scallions.

**3** Make either dressing by combining the ingredients in a small bowl and stirring into the pasta salad to coat the ingredients. Sprinkle the parsley and pine nuts, if using, and serve at once, or chill until required.

✳ **Serve** *with tomato salad or a simple leaf salad.*

✳ **Refrigerate** *in an airtight container for 24 hours without the pine nuts.*

# Carrot and raisin salad

This delicious carrot salad contains juicy segments of orange to boost your baby's vitamin A and C levels. The raisins also provide a sweet contrast that your baby will enjoy.

 10 mins   2 toddler and 3 adult portions

## ingredients

10oz (300g) **carrots**, peeled
or scrubbed, trimmed,
and finely grated
1¾oz (50g) **raisins**
1 large **orange**
1 tbsp **poppy seeds** (optional)
1 tbsp chopped **parsley**

For the dressing:
1 tbsp **olive oil**
1 tbsp **lime juice**
1 tsp **honey**

## method

**1** In a large bowl, mix together the carrots and raisins. Using a sharp knife, peel the orange. Holding the orange over the bowl to catch any drips, cut away the flesh of each segment, halve, and add to the salad. Stir in the poppy seeds, if using, and parsley.

**2** Meanwhile, make the dressing by whisking together the ingredients. Pour over the salad, stir, and chill until required.

＊Serve *with barbequed meat, lasagnas, and other family meals.*
＊Refrigerate *in an airtight container for 24 hours.*
＊Variations: *Add grated beet or ½ red bell pepper instead of the orange.*

# Chicken korma

Mild kormas can contain cream, nuts, coconut, or yogurt. This one uses almonds and coconut and is a delicious family meal. Curry powders and pastes are a surprisingly good source of iron.

 10 mins  20–25 mins  1 toddler and 3 adult portions

Chicken korma

## ingredients

1 tbsp **vegetable oil**
1 medium **onion**,
finely chopped
2 **garlic cloves**, finely chopped
14oz (400g) boneless, skinless
**chicken breasts**, cut into
¾in (2cm) cubes

3 tbsp **korma curry
powder**
1¾oz (50g) almond flour
2 tbsp **coconut milk**
1 heaping tbsp chopped
**cilantro**

## method

**1** Heat the oil in a large saucepan and gently cook the onion and garlic for 7–8 minutes, or until just softened and lightly browned. Add the chicken and cook over low to medium heat, stirring frequently, until the chicken is just cooked on the outside.

**2** Add the curry powder and mix well, cooking for about 1 minute. Stir in the almond flour, 1 cup water, and coconut

milk, and bring the mixture to a simmering point. Stir, cover, and simmer for 10–15 minutes, or until the chicken is cooked through.

**3** Sprinkle over the cilantro, stir through, and remove from the heat. Let cool slightly before serving.

＊Serve *with brown basmati rice, naan, and green vegetables or wilted spinach.*
＊Refrigerate *in an airtight container for up to 24 hours.*

# Chicken stir fry

To retain nutrients and keep vegetables crisp, have everything ready before you cook. Use vegetable, sunflower, or corn oil, not olive oil, which smokes with high temperatures. You can change ingredients to suit your family.

 10 mins     10 mins    ⬤ 1 toddler and 3 adult portions

## ingredients

2 tbsp **vegetable oil**
9oz (250g) boneless, skinless **chicken breasts**, cut into strips
5½oz (150g) **snow peas**, trimmed and sliced into ¼in (5mm) pieces
1 large **red** or **orange bell pepper**, cut into slices

7oz (200g) **bean sprouts**
4 **scallions**, trimmed and finely sliced
1in (3cm) piece of **fresh ginger**, finely grated
2 **garlic cloves**, crushed
2 tbsp reduced-salt **soy sauce**
2 tbsp **dry sherry**

## method

**1** Heat 1 tablespoon of the oil in a non-stick or well-seasoned wok and, over high heat, stir fry the chicken for 2–3 minutes, or until it is white and cooked through. Remove from the pan and keep warm.

**2** Add the remaining oil and stir fry all the remaining ingredients, except the soy sauce

and sherry, for 2–3 minutes, or until they remain just crispy. If the vegetables begin to stick, add 1–2 tablespoons of water.

**3** Return the chicken to the pan, stir in with the soy sauce and sherry, and serve hot with noodles or rice.

✴ *Not suitable for storing.*

✴ *Variations: You can use strips of pork or turkey breast instead of chicken. Use similar quantities of finely sliced carrot or white cabbage instead of the bean sprouts or snow peas.*

*Chicken stir fry*

# Pork with plums

Pork loin is a lean tender cut, suitable for pan-frying or broiling, making a succulent partner to this spicy plum sauce. Pork is particularly rich in vitamin B1.

 15 mins     20 mins     1–2 toddler and 3–4 adult portions

## ingredients

1 tbsp **vegetable oil**, plus extra for brushing
2 **red onions**, finely sliced
3 **garlic cloves**, chopped
2in (5cm) **fresh ginger**, peeled and cut into fine matchsticks

1 tsp **ground allspice**
9oz (250g) **plums**, pitted and quartered
1 tbsp **muscavado sugar**
1lb 2oz (500g) **pork loin** (tenderloin)

## method

**1** Heat the oil and sauté the onion and garlic for about 1 minute, stirring frequently.

**2** Add the ginger, spice, plums, sugar, and ⅔ cup water, and allow to simmer gently for 10 minutes, or until the plums are softened. Let stand while you prepare the pork.

**3** Preheat the oven to 300°F (150°C).

**4** Cut the pork into ½in (1cm) slices and brush lightly with the oil. Broil in batches under a broiler for 3–4 minutes each side, then transfer to a covered dish in the oven while you finish broiling. Serve with the plum sauce.

✴ **Serve** *with boiled rice and steamed or stir-fried green vegetables.*

✴ *The sauce may be refrigerated for 24 hours or frozen when cooled. The cooked pork is not suitable for storing.*

# Lamb and prune tagine

Lamb is rich in iron and zinc, and the delicious spices and succulent fruit make this a popular family meal. If you like a hot tagine, you can add a couple of dried chiles, but remove these before serving.

 15 mins    1¾–2 hours    2 toddler and 3 adult portions   ❄

## ingredients

2 tbsp **vegetable oil**
14oz (400g) lean leg or
  shoulder of **lamb**, cut
  into ¾in (2cm) cubes
2 medium **onions**,
  chopped
2 **garlic cloves**, crushed
3 tsp **ground cumin**
  (see tip)
1 tsp **ground cinnamon**

2 cups well-diluted hot
  **vegetable or lamb stock**
2 tbsp **tomato paste**
2 **lime leaves**
5½oz (150g) dried
  **prunes**, halved, if large
2 tbsp chopped
  **cilantro**
**couscous,** or **natural
  yogurt**, to serve
  (optional)

## method

**1** Preheat the oven to 325°F (170°C). Heat the oil in a non-stick saucepan, add the meat in batches, and stir fry until browned.

**2** Add the onions and cook for another 3 minutes, or until starting to soften. Stir in the garlic and spices and cook for another minute, then pour in

the hot stock. Stir in the purée, lime leaves, and prunes. Transfer to a flameproof casserole, cover, and cook for 1 hour.

**3** Remove from the oven, stir, and return for 30–45 minutes, or until the lamb is really tender.

**4** Remove the lime leaves and stir in the cilantro.

✳ **Serve** *with couscous (if you wish add parsely, lemon zest, and currants), a green leaf salad or steamed green beans.*
✳ **Refrigerate** *for up to 48 hours or freeze on the day of cooking when cool. To defrost, refrigerate overnight and reheat until piping hot.*
✳ **Tip:** *For more flavor, toast cumin seeds in a hot dry pan for a few seconds. Cool, then grind.*

# Moussaka

This popular dish with eggplant, ground lamb, and an egg-enriched sauce can be varied by using beef or soy protein. The eggplant in this version is lightly brushed with oil and broiled rather than fried to keep the fat content down.

 15 mins    1 hour    2 toddler and 4 adult portions   ❄

## ingredients

1 tbsp **vegetable oil**, plus
  extra for greasing
1 large **onion**, finely chopped
2 **garlic cloves**, crushed
10oz (300g) lean **ground lamb**
½ tsp **ground cinnamon**
2 **bay leaves**
2 cups **tomato purée**
2 medium **eggplants**

For the sauce
2 tbsp **flour**
1¼ cups **milk**
1 tbsp **unsalted butter**
  or **olive oil spread**
2 **eggs**, beaten
**black pepper**, to taste
¾oz (20g) **hard cheese**,
  such as Parmesan
grated **nutmeg**

## method

**1** Preheat the oven to 400°F (200°C). Grease a 2-quart (2-liter) flameproof dish.

**2** Heat some oil in a large non-stick saucepan, add the onion and garlic, and cook for 5 minutes over medium heat. Add the lamb and cook until browned, breaking up the lamb with a wooden spoon.

**3** Add the cinnamon, bay leaves, and tomato purée and bring to a simmer. Stir, cover, and simmer for 10–15 minutes. Take off the heat and remove the bay leaves.

**4** Meanwhile, trim the eggplant stems and cut lengthwise into slices roughly ½in (1cm) thick. Brush lightly with oil and place under a broiler to soften and brown a little. Remove

from the heat and let cool slightly.

**5** Make the sauce by mixing together the flour and a little milk in a saucepan over a low heat, or bowl if you prefer to make it in the microwave. When smooth, add the remaining milk and butter. Heat, stirring often, until the sauce thickens. (In the microwave, cook on high and stir every 40 seconds.) Cool a little before stirring in the eggs, pepper, and cheese.

**6** Place a third of the lamb at the bottom of the dish and top with half the eggplant. Repeat, finishing with the lamb. Pour the sauce over the dish and grate nutmeg on top. Bake for 25–30 minutes, or until golden brown.

✳ **Serve** *with fresh crusty bread, Whole grain salad (see p212), steamed green vegetables or Sugar snap and apple salad (see p210).*
✳ **Refrigerate** *for up to 24 hours or freeze on the day of cooking when cooled.*
✳ **Variations:** *Lean beef or soy products, such as quorn, can be used instead of the lamb.*

# Beef goulash

Goulash is a great source of iron and zinc and makes a nutritious family meal, served with noodles or mashed potatoes. Traditionally made with beef, onions, and paprika, goulash can also be made with other vegetables and spices. Paprika varies in strength; for this recipe it is best to use mild or sweet smoked paprika.

 10 mins    1¾–2 hours    1 toddler and 3–4 adult portions   ❄

## ingredients

- 2 tbsp **vegetable oil**
- 1 medium **onion**, halved and sliced
- 2 **garlic cloves,** crushed
- 1 tbsp **all-purpose flour** or **cornstarch**
- 1–2 tsp **mild** or **sweet smoked paprika**
- 14oz (400g) **lean beef stew meat**, cut into ¾in (2cm) cubes
- 1 cup **water** or diluted **beef stock**
- 2 medium **green bell peppers,** cut into large pieces
- 1 x 14oz (400g) can chopped **tomatoes** in juice

## method

**1** Preheat the oven to 325°F (160°C).

**2** Heat the oil in a large flameproof casserole pan and cook the onion for 5 minutes, or until lightly browned. Stir in the garlic and cook for about 1 minute.

**3** Coat the meat with flour by placing the flour, paprika, and meat in a clean plastic food bag and shaking. Pour the floured meat and

any remaining seasoned flour into the pan and stir around briefly.

**4** Add the water or stock, peppers, and tomatoes, and bring slowly to a simmering point, stirring frequently.

**5** Cover and transfer to the oven and cook for 1½ hours. Check and stir, and return to the oven until the meat is really tender.

＊Serve *with low-fat sour cream or natural yogurt, noodles, potatoes, or green vegetables.*

＊Refrigerate *in an airtight container for up to two days or freeze when cooled. Defrost overnight in the fridge, and, ideally, reheat in a microwave oven until piping hot before use.*

Natural yogurt

Beef goulash

# Mild chili con carne

*Mild chili con carne*

This simple family dish can be made in bulk and frozen. It provides iron, zinc, fiber, and a host of B vitamins. Keep it mild, adding your own chilli sauce afterward if you like.

 10 mins   40–45 mins   2 toddler and 4 adult portions

## ingredients

2 tbsp **vegetable oil**
1 medium **onion**, finely chopped
1lb (450g) **extra lean ground beef**
1 **garlic clove**, crushed
1 large **red bell pepper**, seeded and diced
½ tsp **sweet smoked paprika**

1 tsp **ground cumin**
1 x 14oz (400g) can chopped **tomatoes**
2 tbsp **tomato paste**
1 x 14oz (400g) can **red kidney beans** in water, rinsed and drained
¾ cup **water** or diluted **beef stock**
**chili** or **piri piri sauce** (optional)

## method

**1** Heat the oil in a large non-stick saucepan. Add the onion and cook, stirring, over medium heat for 2–3 minutes.

**2** Stir in the beef and garlic and cook for 5 minutes, or until the meat is browned, breaking up the beef with a wooden spoon. Add the remaining ingredients and bring to a simmering point.

**3** Reduce the heat, cover, and cook for 30–35 minutes, stirring occasionally. Add more water if it's too thick and begins to stick to the pan.

**4** When the sauce becomes thick, moist, and juicy, it is cooked. Remove your child's portion, and if you want to add some heat to your portion, add the extra chili seasoning.

✳ **Serve** *with plain boiled rice, a baked potato, or wrap in a tortilla with shredded lettuce.*

✳ **Refrigerate** *in an airtight container for up to 48 hours or freeze when cooled.*

# Lasagna al forno

A succulent iron-rich dish, lasagna is a worldwide classic. You can replace the meat with textured soy protein.

 15 mins   60–80 mins   2 toddler and 4 adult portions

## ingredients

For the ragu:
1 tbsp **vegetable oil**, plus extra for greasing
1 small **onion**, finely chopped
1 **garlic clove**, crushed
14oz (400g) **lean ground steak**
½ **red bell pepper**, finely chopped
14oz (400g) can chopped **tomatoes** in juice
2 tbsp **tomato paste**

¼ cup **red wine** or **water**
2 **bay leaves**
1 tbsp chopped **thyme**
For the white sauce:
¼ cup **all-purpose flour**
2 cups **milk**
2 tbsp **olive oil spread** or **butter**
**nutmeg**, to grate
5½oz (150g) **lasagna sheets**
1¾oz (50g) **Cheddar cheese**

## method

**1** Preheat the oven to 375°F (190°C). Lightly grease a lasagna pan.

**2** Heat the oil in a non-stick saucepan; gently cook the onion, garlic, and steak, breaking up the meat with a wooden spoon until the steak is separated.

**3** Add the pepper; cook, stirring frequently, until the vegetables are soft and the meat brown. Add the tomatoes, paste, water or wine, bay leaves, and thyme, and simmer. Stir, cover, and cook for 15–20 minutes, stirring a little. Remove the bay leaves.

**4** Meanwhile, make the sauce. Whisk the flour, milk, and butter in a saucepan over medium heat until the sauce bubbles and thickens. Cook for 1 minute. Grate in the nutmeg.

**5** Pour ⅓ the ragu into the dish, add a layer of lasagna sheets, and spread a quarter of the sauce on top. Repeat until you've used all the ragu and lasagna, then add the cheese to the remaining sauce and pour over the top. Bake for 40–45 minutes, or until the sauce is bubbling, golden brown, and the pasta soft when pierced with a sharp knife. Stand for 5 minutes then serve.

✳ **Serve** *with a salad and crusty bread.*

✳ **Refrigerate** *overnight covered in plastic wrap or freeze in an airtight container when cooled*

# Salmon in filo pastry

Wrapping salmon in filo keeps in the moisture and looks great. This makes a handy picnic food served cold.

 5 mins  20 mins  2 toddler and 1 adult portions

## ingredients

- 2 medium **salmon fillets**, preferably skinless
- 4–5 sheets of **phyllo dough**
- **juice** of ½ **lemon** or **lime**
- 1 tbsp chopped **parsley**
- **vegetable oil**, for brushing

## method

**1** Preheat the oven to 400°F (200°C).

**2** Remove the salmon's skin, if not skinned already, and check for bones by running your finger over the flesh; remove any you find. Cut off a thumb-sized piece for your baby's portion.

**3** Lay a sheet of phyllo dough on a clean surface; spray or brush with oil. Place 1 baby piece of salmon near the short end of the pastry rectangle, squeeze over lemon, and add a little parsley. Roll the dough over to cover the fish and tuck in the sides. Once you have a little parcel, put this on a lightly oiled baking sheet and spray or brush with oil.

**4** Make 2 baby portions, then repeat for the adult portions. If the salmon is visible, use 1 more sheet, oiling first so it sticks. Bake for 20 minutes, or until golden brown. Cool a little before serving.

＊**Serve** *hot with mixed vegetables, new potatoes, or salad.*

＊**Refrigerate** *in an airtight container for up to 24 hours.*

＊**Variations:** *Add chopped scallions, and/or slices of red bell pepper, or asparagus pieces in season.*

# Tuna noodle casserole

Each family has its own version of this dish, which is a meal in itself. It's a great standby as most of the ingredients are pantry basics.

 20 mins  15–30 mins  2 toddler and 3 adult portions

## ingredients

- 9oz (250g) **penne pasta**
- **vegetable oil** (optional)
- 3½oz (100g) **peas**, defrosted
- 3½oz (100g) **corn kernels**, frozen defrosted, or canned in water
- 2 x 6½oz (185g) cans of **tuna** in water, drained

For the sauce:
- 2 cups **whole milk**
- ¼ cup **all-purpose flour**
- 2 tbsp **butter** or **olive oil spread**
- 1 tsp **mustard** (optional)
- 2 tbsp **tomato paste**
- 1¾oz (50g) **Cheddar cheese**

## method

**1** Cook the pasta in boiling water until just tender and drain. Return to the pan, cover, and add a drizzle of oil, if needed, to prevent from sticking to the pan.

**2** Meanwhile, make the sauce by placing the milk, flour, and butter in a large pan and whisking over medium heat until it bubbles and thickens. Reduce the heat and cook for 2 minutes. Stir in the mustard, if using, tomato paste, and half the cheese.

**3** Add the peas, corn, tuna, and pasta, and stir well. Pour into a flameproof dish, sprinkle with the remaining cheese, and put under a preheated broiler for 4–5 minutes, or until the cheese bubbles and browns. Or place in a preheated 350°F (180°C) oven and bake for 15–20 minutes. Cool for 1–2 minutes before serving.

＊**Serve** *with additional green vegetables or a side salad.*

＊**Refrigerate** *for 24 hours. Reheat until piping hot, preferably in a microwave to prevent it from drying out.*

Tuna noodle casserole

# Vegetarian lasagna

These come in many forms, some using lentils or beans, others soy protein. This uses a type of vitamin-C rich ratatouille that makes a delicious, moist lasagna.

 20 mins  70–75 mins 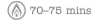 2 toddler and 4 adult portions

## ingredients

2 tbsp **olive oil**, plus extra for greasing
1 medium **onion**, halved and sliced
2 **garlic cloves**, chopped
1 medium **red** or **yellow pepper**, cut into chunks
1 medium **eggplant**, cut into ½in (1cm) cubes
1 medium **zucchini**, sliced
2 x 14oz (400g) cans chopped **tomatoes**
1 tbsp **mixed herbs**, such as oregano/thyme
5½oz (150g) **oven-ready lasagna noodles**

For the sauce:
¼ cup **all-purpose flour**
2 cups **milk**
2 tbsp **unsalted butter** or **olive oil spread**
grated nutmeg
2½oz (75g) sharp **Cheddar cheese**, grated

## method

**1** Preheat the oven to 375°F (190°C). Lightly grease a large lasagna dish.

**2** Heat the oil in a pan. Gently cook the onion and garlic for 5 minutes, until just soft. Add the pepper; cook for 2–3 minutes.

**3** Stir in the eggplant, zucchini, tomatoes, and herbs. Bring the mixture to a simmering point, stir, and cover. Cook for 20 minutes while you make the sauce, stirring occasionally.

**4** Whisk the flour and milk in a saucepan and add the butter. Heat, whisking continuously, until the sauce bubbles and thickens. Cook for 1 minute, and grate in some nutmeg.

**5** Pour or spoon around a third of the mixture into the dish, add a layer of lasagna sheets, and spread a quarter of the sauce on top. Repeat until you have used all the vegetables and lasagna, then add the cheese to the rest of the sauce, and pour over the top.

**6** Bake for 40–45 minutes, or until the sauce is bubbling, golden, and the pasta soft when pierced with a sharp knife. Stand for 5 minutes before serving.

✳ **Serve** *with a green salad, Whole grain salad (see p212), or crusty bread.*

✳ **Refrigerate** *in an airtight container for up to 24 hours or freeze when cooled.*

Vegetarian lasagna

# Vegetable chow mein

A delicious and speedy meal that is full of nutritious vegetables, topped with crunchy cashew nuts.

 5 mins  10 mins  1 toddler and 2 adult portions

## ingredients

9oz (250g) **egg noodles**
1 tbsp **sesame** or **vegetable oil**
2 tbsp **vegetable oil**
2 **garlic cloves**, chopped
1in (3cm) piece **fresh ginger**, finely grated
3½oz (100g) **mushrooms**, sliced
1 **red** or **orange bell pepper**, finely sliced
2 tbsp **dry sherry**
2 tbsp low salt **soy sauce**
1 head **bok choy**, sliced
3½oz (100g) **bean sprouts**, rinsed and well drained
4 **scallions**, in ½in (1cm) slices
3½oz (100g) **cashew nuts**, toasted
1 tbsp chopped **cilantro** (optional)

## method

**1** Cook the noodles according to the pack instructions. Rinse, drain, and toss in the sesame oil to separate them. Put to one side while you cook the stir fry.

**2** Heat the oil in a wok. Add the garlic and ginger, frying briefly, then the mushrooms and pepper.

Stir fry for 2–3 minutes. Add the sherry and soy sauce, quickly followed by the noodles, bok choy, beans prouts, and scallions, stirring continuously. Add 1 tablespoon of water if sticky.

**3** Serve with sprinkled cashews and cilantro, if using.

✳ *Not suitable for storage.*

✳ **Variations:** *Omit or replace the cashews with plain unsalted toasted peanuts.*

# Dealing with choking

**As a new parent** it is a good idea to attend a special baby and child first aid course with a First Aid training organization so that you know what to do if an emergency affects a child in your care. These courses will teach you everything from how to treat cuts and choking to what to do if your child ever loses consciousness. You will learn how to give cardiopulmonary resuscitation (CPR), a combination of chest compressions and rescue breaths, which is a potentially life-saving technique used to treat a child who has stopped breathing.

## How to deal with choking

A baby can choke on small pieces of food or after putting a small object in his or her mouth. Don't intervene if your baby is able to cough as your action could cause the obstruction to move further down the airway, but if he or she becomes distressed and is unable to breathe or make a noise, treat as described below.

- If your baby is distressed, is unable to cry, cough, or breathe, you need to take emergency action to clear her airway. Lay her face down along your thigh and support her head and upper body with one hand. Using the heel of your other hand, give up to five sharp blows to the upper part of her back between the shoulder blades.

- Turn her over so that she is face up along your other leg and check her mouth. If you can clearly see a loose object, remove it carefully with your fingertips. Do not sweep the inside of her mouth with your fingers or feel blindly down her throat as you may push an object further in or damage her throat.

- If the back blows have not cleared the obstruction, try chest thrusts. With the baby lying face up along your leg, support her upper body and head with one hand and give up to five chest thrusts, by pushing down with two fingers of your other hand on the lower part of the breastbone.

- Check quickly after each chest thrust to see if the obstruction has been dislodged. If the obstruction does not clear after three cycles of five back blows and five chest thrusts, call for an ambulance.

- Continue giving cycles of back blows then mouth checks, and chest thrusts then mouth checks until the ambulance arrives.

**Giving back blows** Make sure the baby's head is lower than her body. Keeping your fingers raised, use the heel of your hand to give back blows; make sure the blows fall between her shoulder blades.

**Giving chest thrusts** Place your first two fingers on the lower half of the baby's breastbone; make sure they are not on the ribs. Push inward and downward toward the baby's head.

# Index

baked egg with cheese and tomato 172

hard-boiled egg 69

scrambled eggs 99

## F

family meals 23, 48, 136, 140–141

meal planner 206–209

fast foods 198

fats 14, 16

fiber 13, 18, 198

finger foods 22, 40, 48, 76, 78–79

commercial snack foods 78

fruits 130–131

vegetables 118–119

first meal 42–43

fish 13, 33, 40, 202

cheesy mash with fish and peas 117

cod, pea, and potato 72

creamy salmon and pasta 121

crispy salmon fingers 186

flaked fish 106

Greek baked fish 120

Italian tomato and tuna mash 120

pasta, tuna, and corn salad 212

salmon and dill risotto 186

salmon and sweet potato 72

salmon and sweet potato cakes 121

salmon in filo pastry 218

salmon, yogurt, and cucumber filling 176

sardines on toast 173

simple fish pie 187

sweet potatoes with sardines and peas 117

tuna dip 105

tuna noodle casserole 218

tuna and tomato pizza 179

fish oil supplements 17

folic acid 14, 17

food intolerances 32

freezing and defrosting 27, 58

French toast with fruit 98

fruit 13, 18

dried fruit 78

finger foods 78, 130–131

first fruits 43

orchard fruits breakfast 70

fruit fool 133

fruit juices 25, 47, 200

fruit with chocolate dipping sauce 135

fussy eaters and food refusal 21, 49, 138, 198, 204–205

## GHIK

gluten 32, 33

good eating habits 48, 138, 140

grapes 130, 201

green beans 119

growth and development 14–15

herbal drinks 47

high chairs 30, 31, 42

honey 18, 19

hygiene 26, 27, 31, 80

independent feeding 20, 21, 48, 78, 136

iron 10, 14, 16, 40, 41, 47, 198, 200

iron-deficiency anemia (IDA) 199

kale 43, 201

kiwi fruit 130, 201

banana and kiwi breakfast 97

exotic fruit salad 191

## L

lamb 202

baby's first lamb tagine 115

bulgur wheat with lamb and eggplant 184

herby lamb with vegetables 114

lamb and apricots 75

lamb and prune tagine 215

mini lamb and mint balls 109

moussaka 215

leeks 64, 66

leek and potato soup 180

sweet potato, barley, and leek soup 102

lentils 199, 202

carrot and lentil soup 103

coconut lentil dhal 128

lentil and spinach dhal 128

lentil, tomato, and coriander dhal 73

vegetarian shepherd's pie 189

liver 17, 19, 202

low- and reduced-fat foods 14, 19

lumpy food 22, 40, 76, 136

## MN

mandarin gelatin 192

mangoes 43, 59, 131

exotic fruit salad 191

fruity chicken 112

mango and vanilla breakfast 97

mango ice pops 132

mango smoothie 171

passion fruit and mango dessert 191

mashed food 40, 41, 76

meal planner

stage 1 50–57

stage 2 82–95

stage 3 142–167

meat 13, 28, 40

see also beef; lamb; pork

messy eating 31, 138

milk

allergy 33

breast milk 10, 12, 14, 15, 33, 45

cow's milk 13, 17, 24, 47, 199, 200, 202

formula feeding 12, 14, 15, 45, 47

fortified milks 199, 200

goat and sheep's milk 25

milk to meals 12–13

rice and nut milks 47

soy milk 47

stage 1 weaning 40, 45

stage 2 weaning 76

stage 3 weaning 136

timing milk feeds 76

millet 68

mixed berry frozen yogurt 133

mixed berry smoothie 168

mushrooms

chicken and mushroom casserole 113

mushroom and onion pizza 178

vegetable chow mein 219

nectarines 131, 201

new foods, introducing 40

nutrients 14–17, 198

nuts 19, 33, 202

see also peanut butter

## OP

oats 68

apricot oatmeal 68

banana oatmeal 68

basic oatmeal 98

bircher muesli 98

pear and raisin oat crumble 193

raspberry oatmeal 99

simple muesli 169

oils 25, 198

omega 3 fatty acids 14, 16, 200

organic food 19

overweight 21, 44, 47, 139, 140

pancakes 169

pantry basics 24–25

papaya 62, 131

parsnips 43, 62, 65, 119

butterbean, parsnip, and sweet potato 73

pasta 18, 25, 28, 76, 79, 201, 203

chicken and pasta with creamy sauce 183

creamy avocado pasta 188

creamy salmon and pasta 121

lasagna al forno 217

macaroni and cheese 125

pasta, tuna, and corn salad 212

tuna noodle casserole 218

vegetarian lasagna 219

yummy veggie sauce with pasta 122

peaches 43, 131, 201

baked spiced peach 190

peach chutney 182

spicy peach breakfast 96

peanut butter

fruity couscous with peanut sauce 189

spicy peanut dip 111

toast and peanut butter 101

pears 43, 59, 66, 67, 130, 202

blueberry and pear breakfast 97

pear and raisin oat crumble 193

yogurt with cinnamon and pear 67

peas 43, 60, 65, 199

cheesy mash with fish and peas 117

cod, pea, and potato 72

pea and mint soup 181

sugar snap and apple salad 210

sweet potatoes with sardines and peas 117

tuna noodle casserole 218

peppers 119

ratatouille 124

roasted Mediterranean vegetable dip 107

turkey and red pepper patties 184

# Useful resources

www.healthychildren.org
A website from the American Academy of Pediatrics on childhood health

www.eatright.org/kids/
Scientifically-based nutritional information for families

www.chopchopmag.org
An online cooking magazine for families

www.letsmove.gov
National movement to get kids to eat healthier and exercise more

www.actionforhealthykids.org
Helping parents understand how to provide nutritional meals for their kids

www.babycenter.com
Expert advice on all things baby

www.askdrsears.com
Holistic approach to feeding your baby

www.foodallergy.org
Information and advice about food allergies

www.nutrition.org
Provides the latest research on nutrition

www.usda.gov
Information about food safety issues as well as nutrition guidelines

www.choosemyplate.gov
Practical information and tips to help build a healthy diet based on USDA dietary guidelines

www.vrg.org
Information, recipes, and guidance for vegetarian and vegan families

# Acknowledgments

## Author's acknowledgments

Thank you Dorling Kindersley for giving me the opportunity to write a book that combines both my experience in infant nutrition and creativity in the kitchen. I hope that for readers it provides an authoritative guide to feeding in the early years, giving practical advice, delicious nutritious recipes, and clear information.

I'd like to acknowledge the team I've worked with on this book, whose enthusiasm and commitment has been exemplary. So thank you Claire for being a great editor and Harriet for bringing the pages to life with your beautiful images and creativity. Thank you too to Anna for her "big picture" perspective, and Lizzie for her efficiency behind the scenes.

Thanks also are due to my family whose meals have been somewhat unusual while the recipes progressed, but who at least were spared stage one recipes!

## Publisher's acknowledgments

DK would like to thank Claire Wedderburn-Maxwell for proofreading; Marie Lorimer for the index; Liz Hippisley for prop styling; Georgie Besterman for food styling; Dr. Su Laurent for consulting on the premature baby spread; and Dr. Carol Cooper for consulting on the allergy spread. Thanks to Collette Sadler for design assistance and Elizabeth Clinton for editorial assistance. All images © Dorling Kindersley. For more information see www.dkimages.com